Nurture your inner Picasso.

Who needs radiation or chemotherapy when you can simply pull out your Crayolas and let the magic happen? Prepare for some serious artistic healing – sarcasm intended.

So go ahead, color your little heart out while those pesky cancer cells retreat in fear of your artistic prowess. And don't forget to calm your mind as well, because clearly that's the secret ingredient for healing a body ravaged by this deadly disease.

I mean, who needs evidence-based treatments and scientific advancements when we have coloring books and deep breathing techniques? While the idea of using coloring books and deep breathing techniques as a sole solution for curing cancer may seem far-fetched and sarcastic, it is important to acknowledge the power of holistic approaches in complementing evidence-based treatments.

Art therapy, including coloring, has been shown to provide emotional support and stress relief. By combining the benefits of both conventional medicine and alternative approaches, we can provide the best possible care for cancer patients.

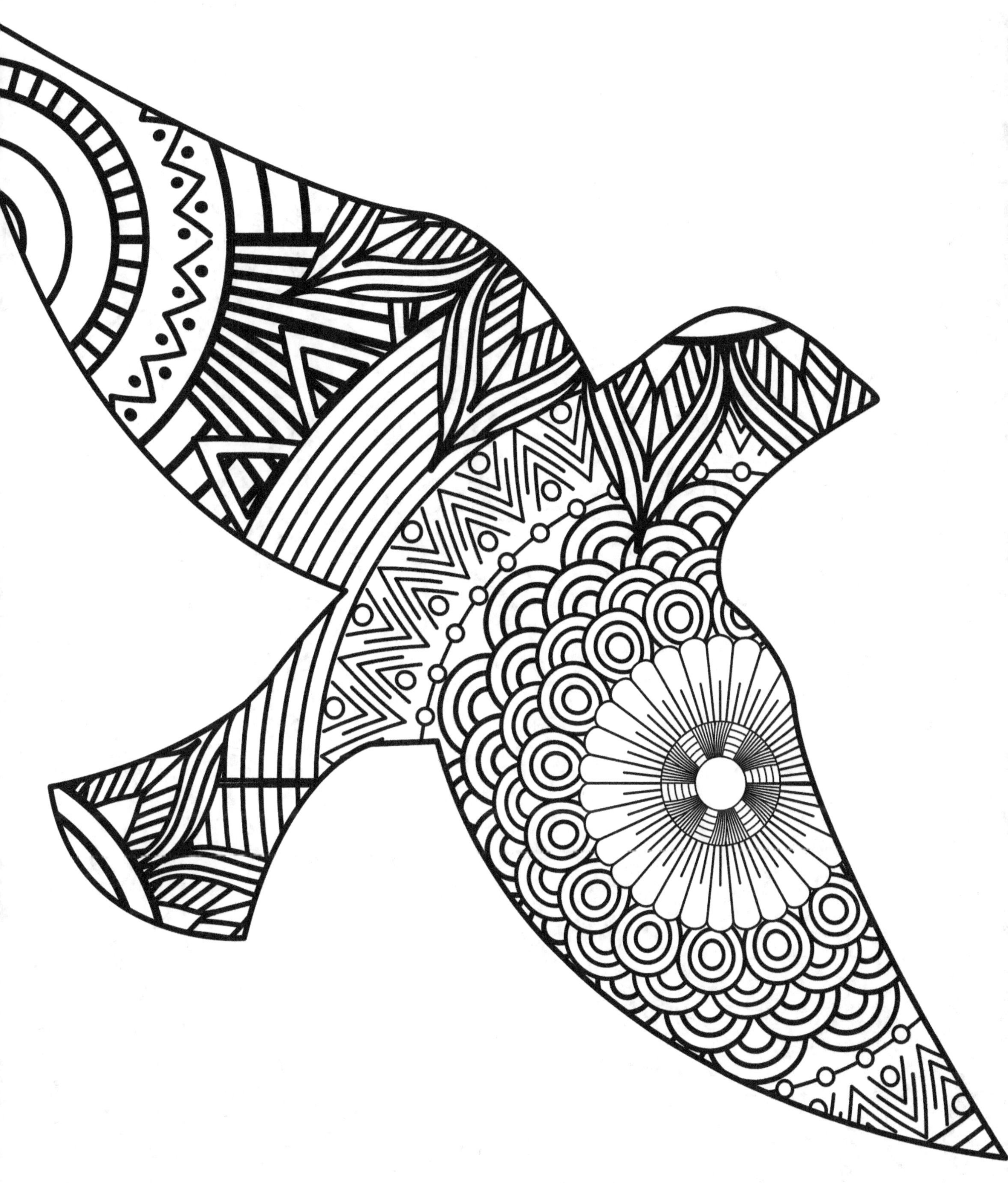

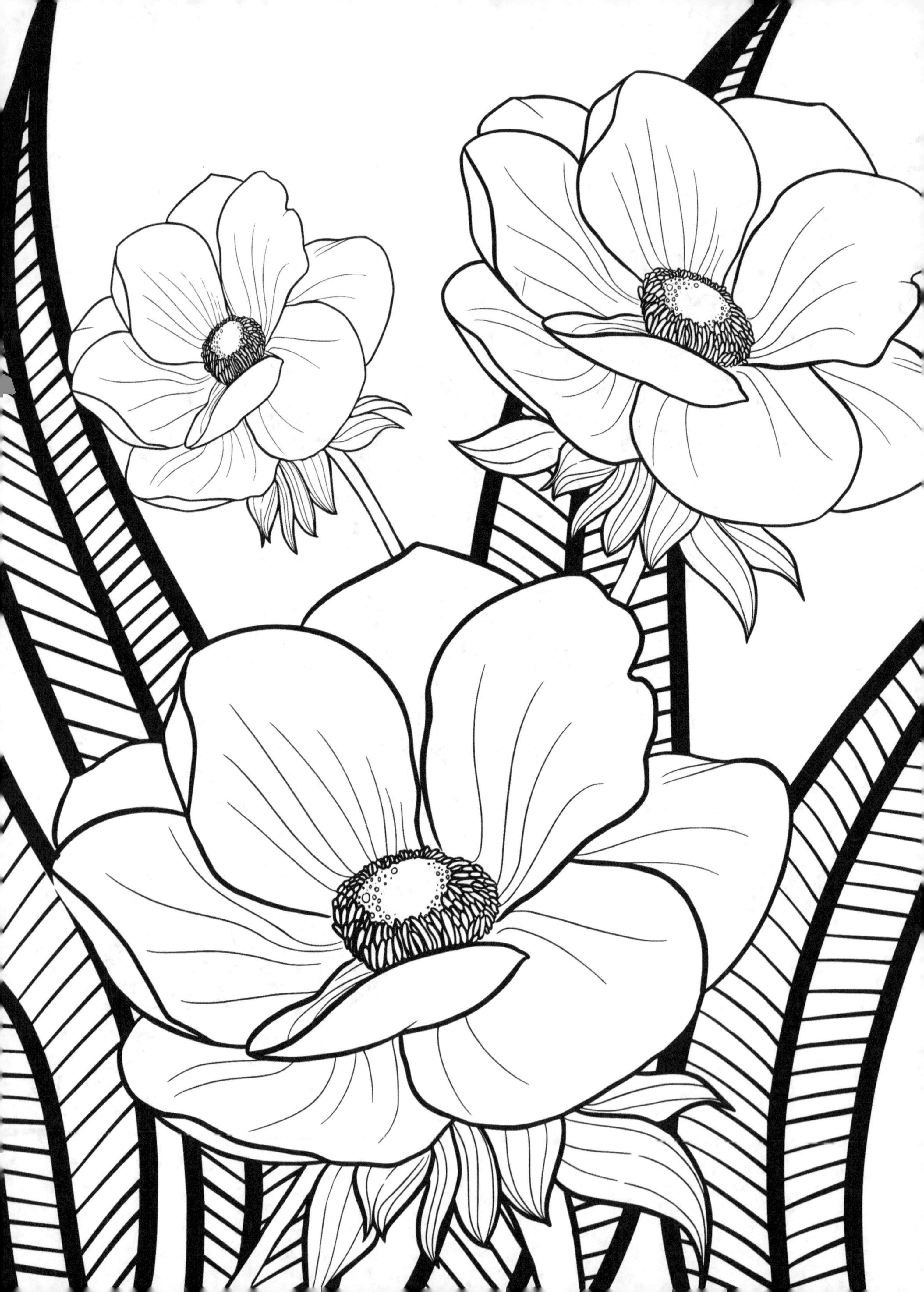

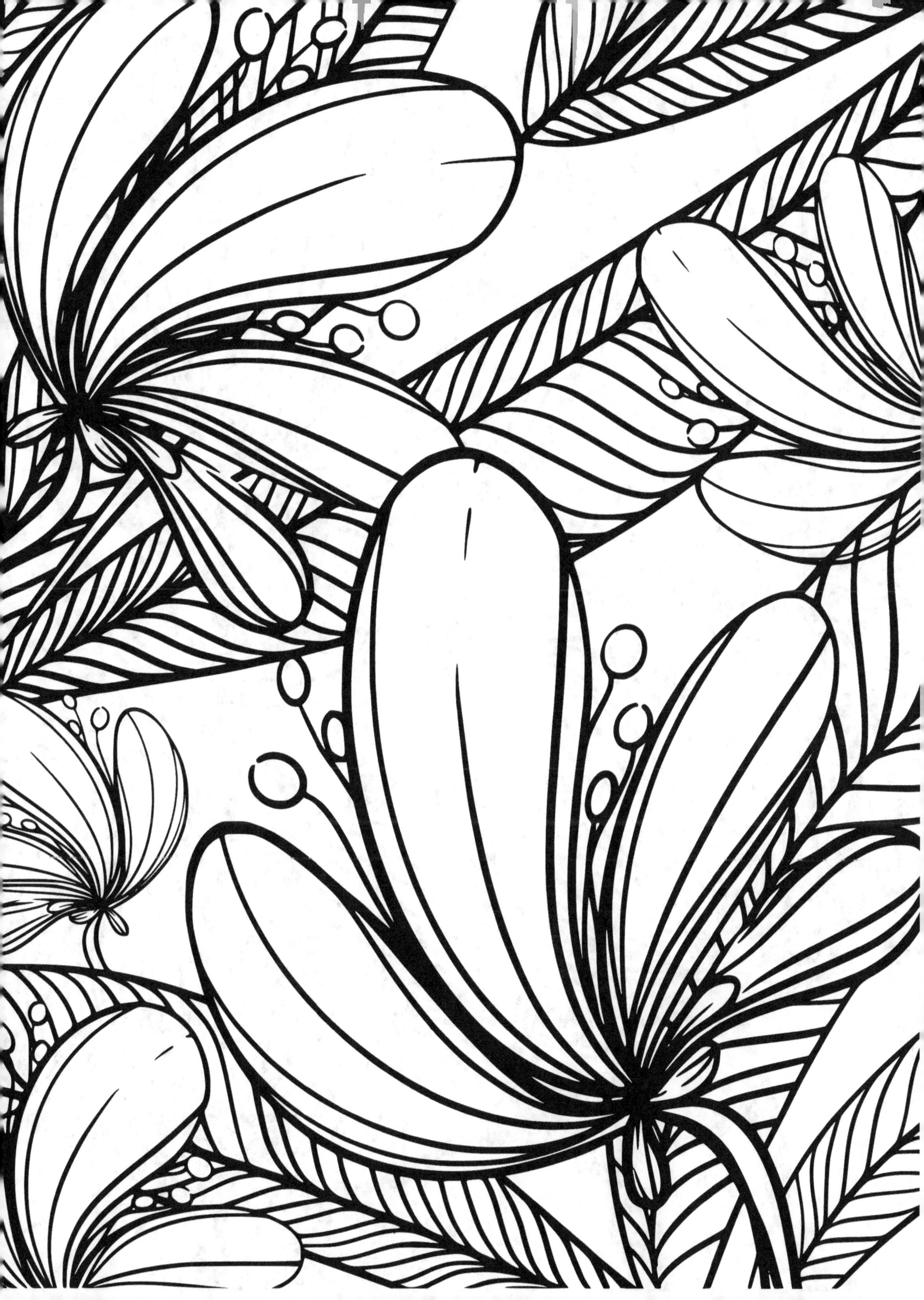

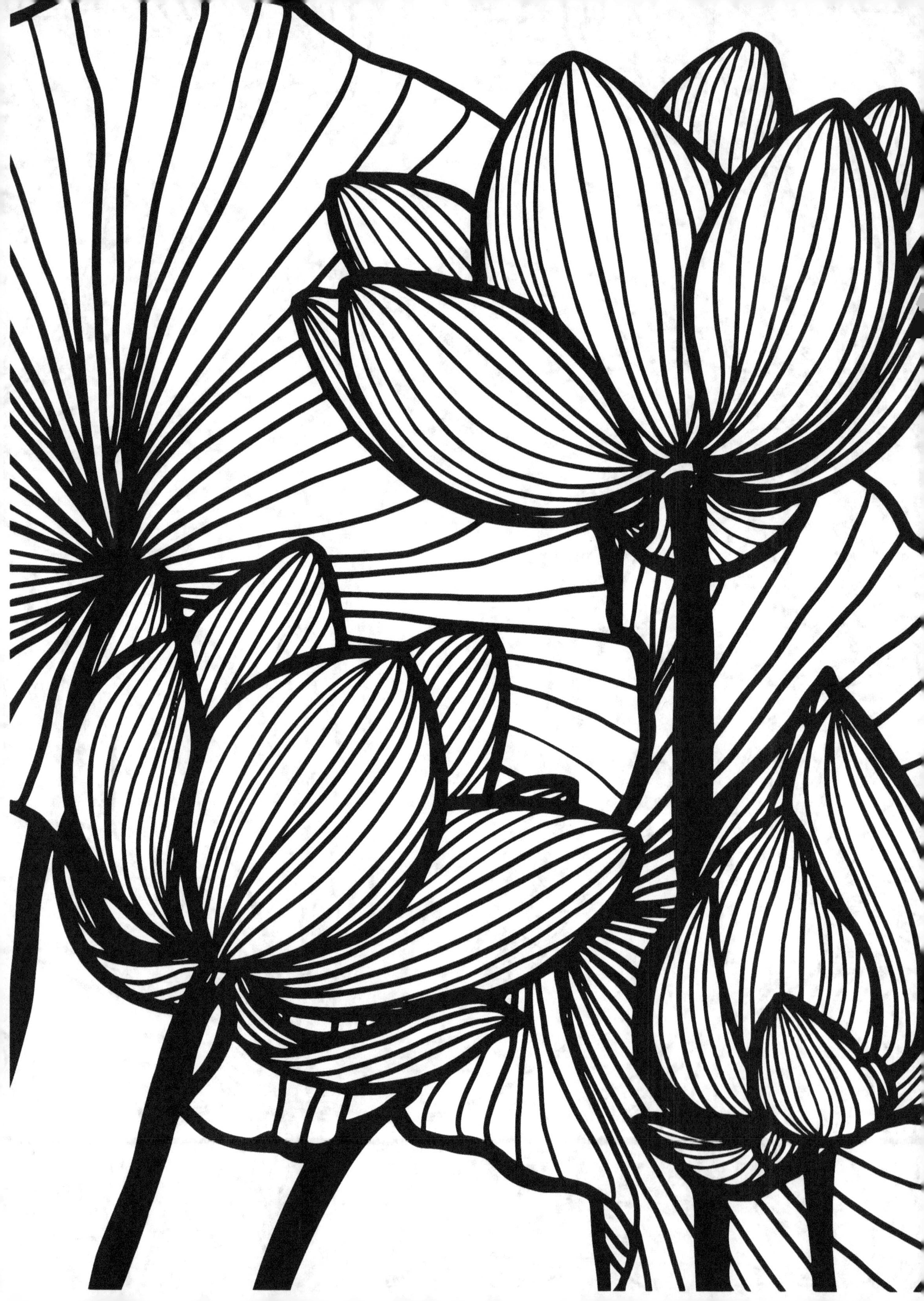

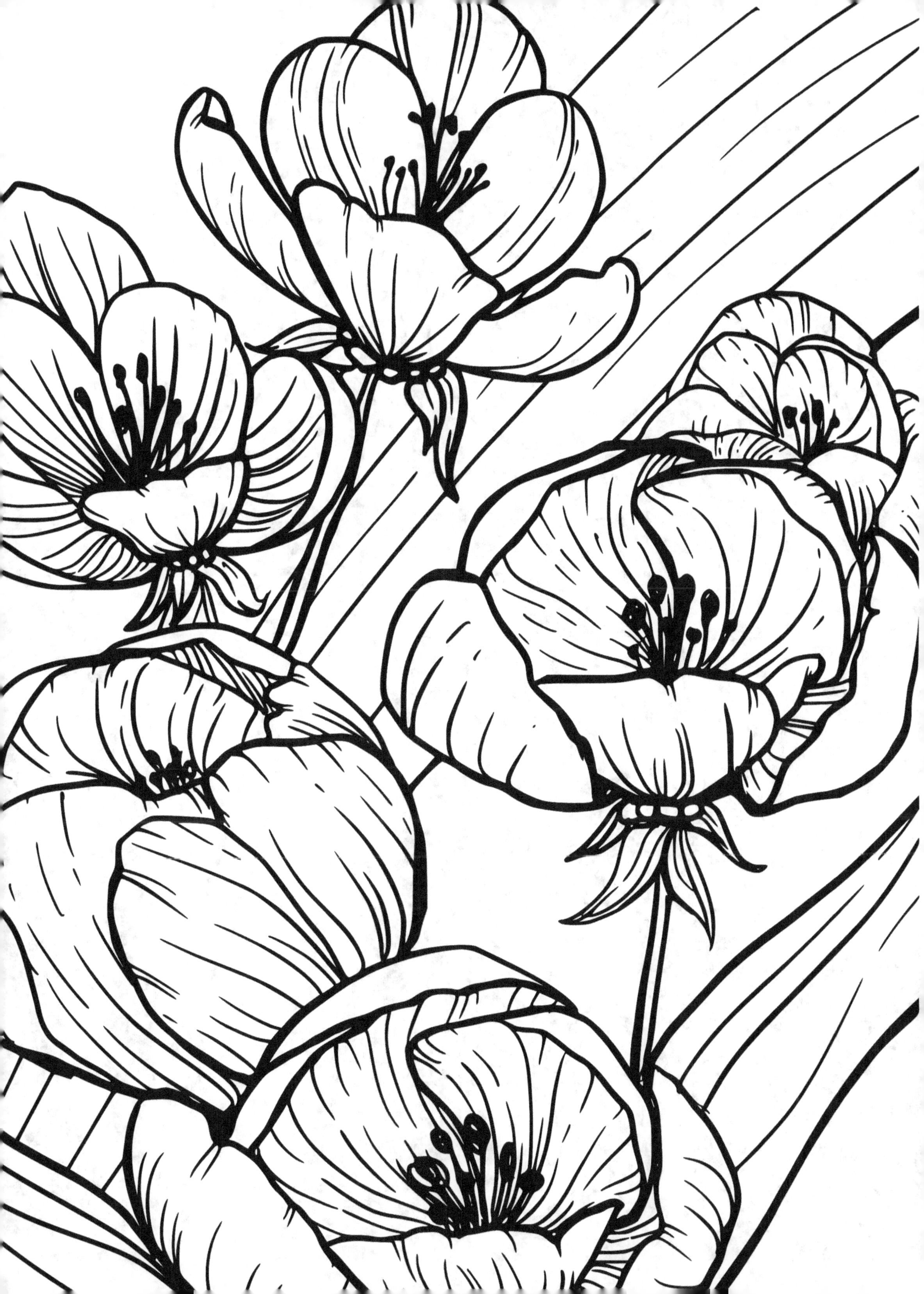

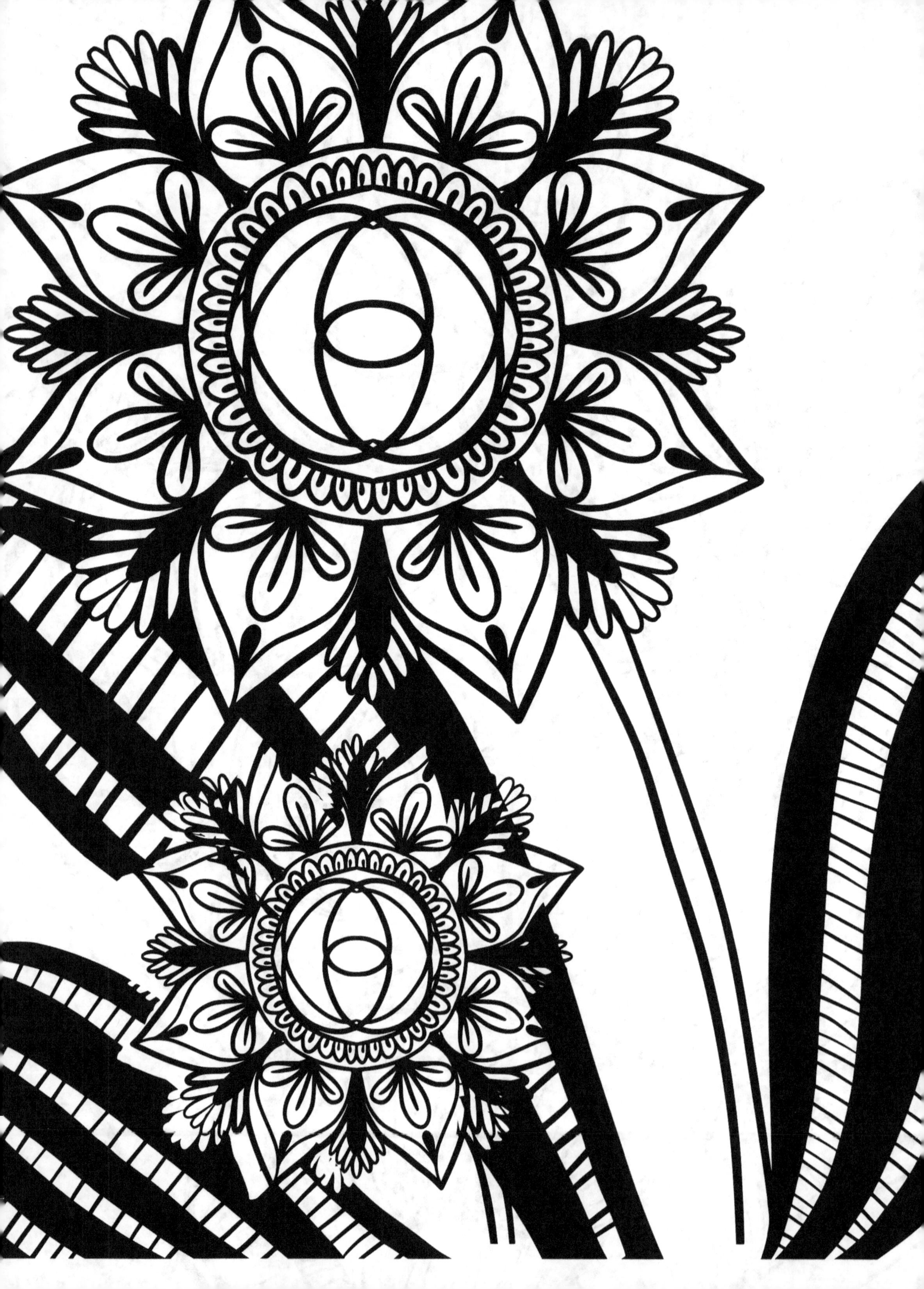

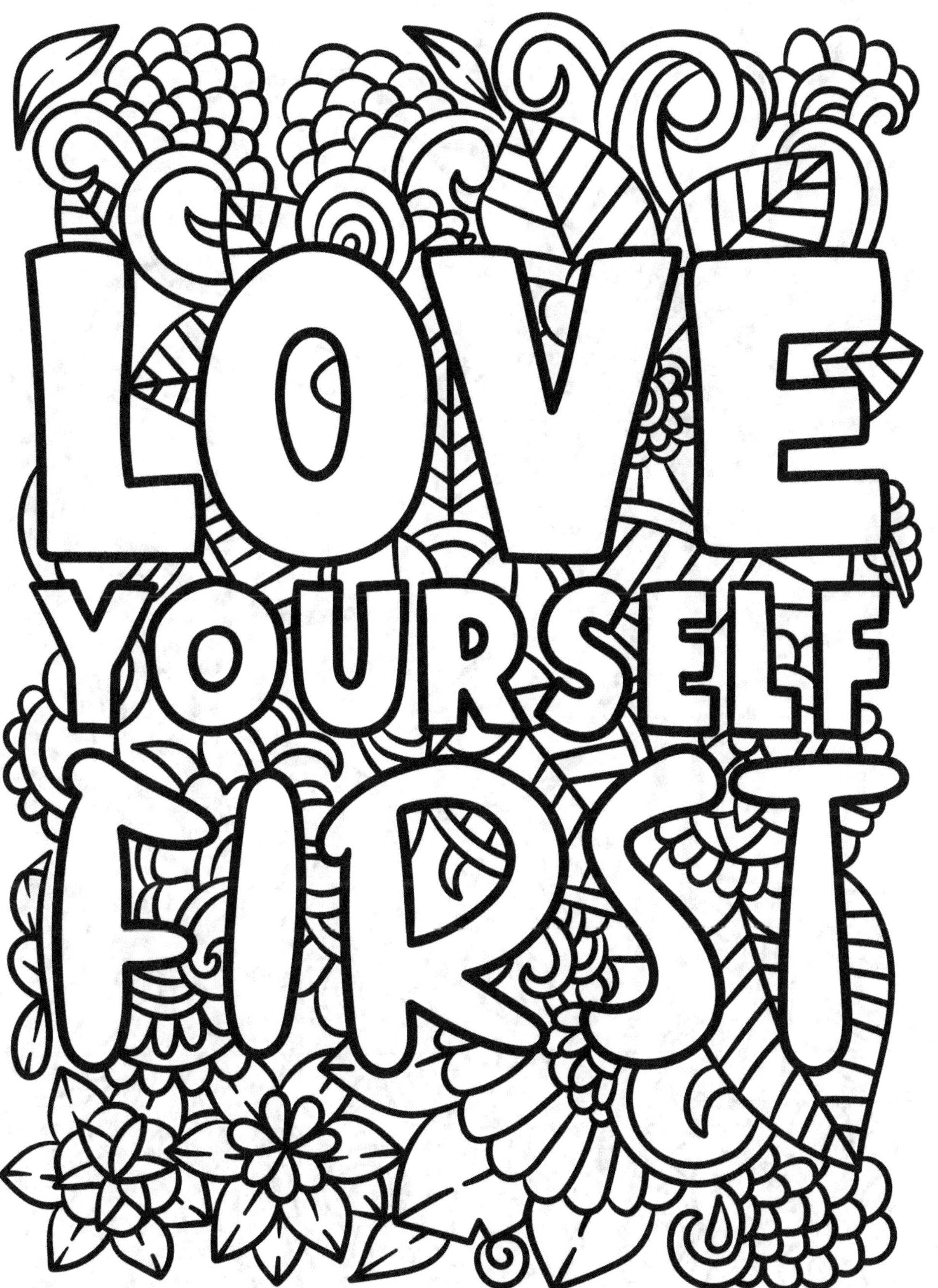

LOVE
YOURSELF
FIRST

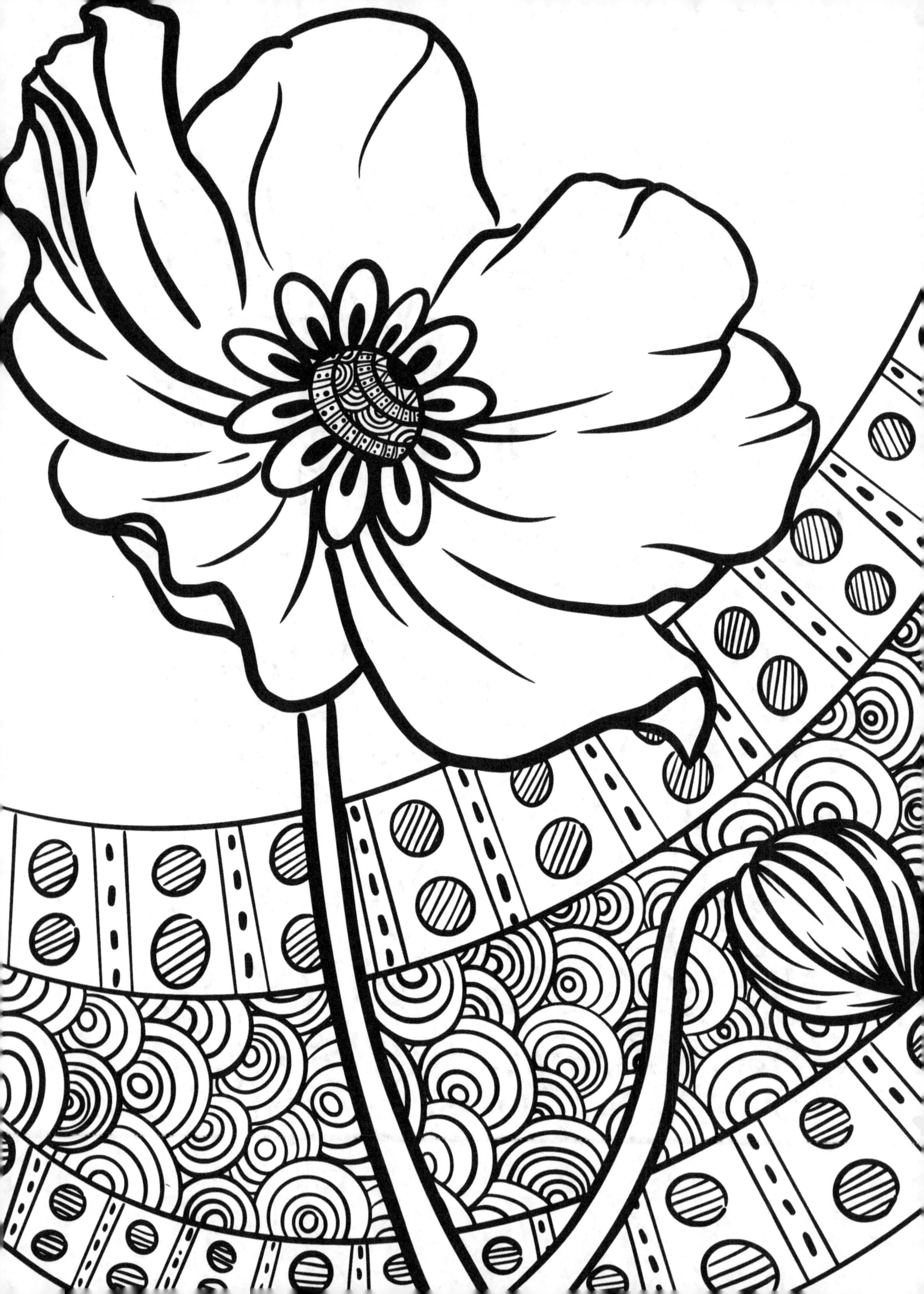

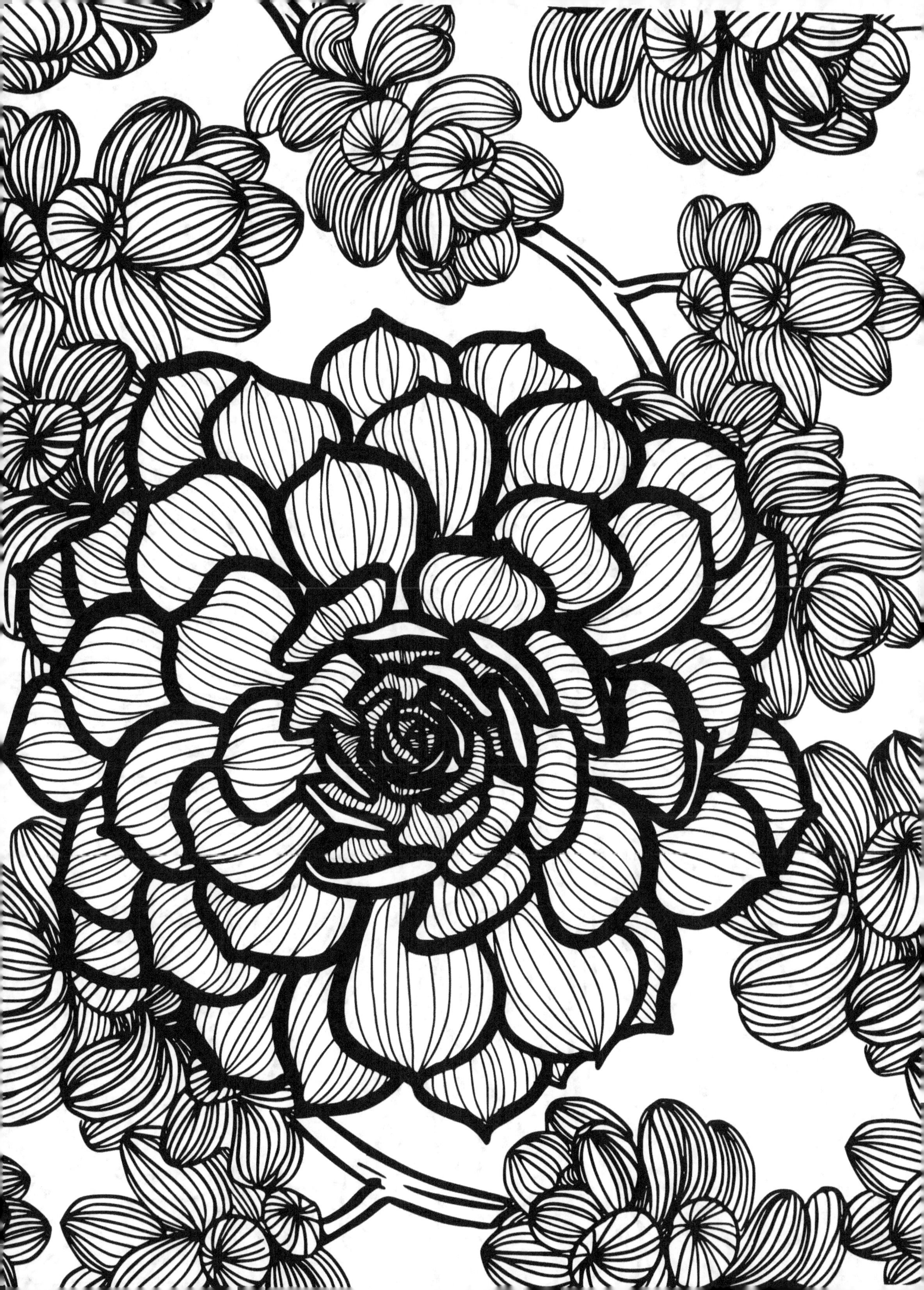

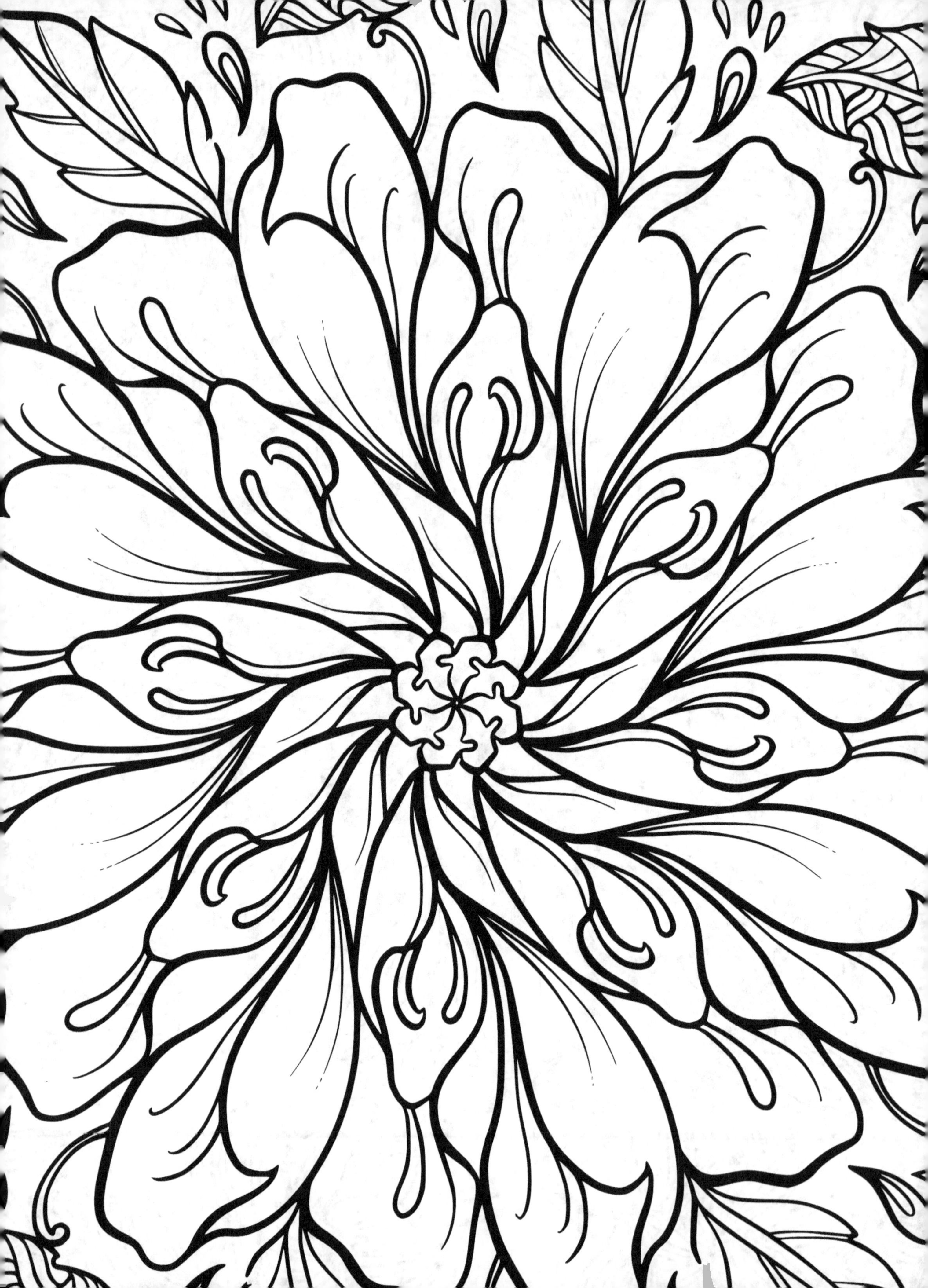

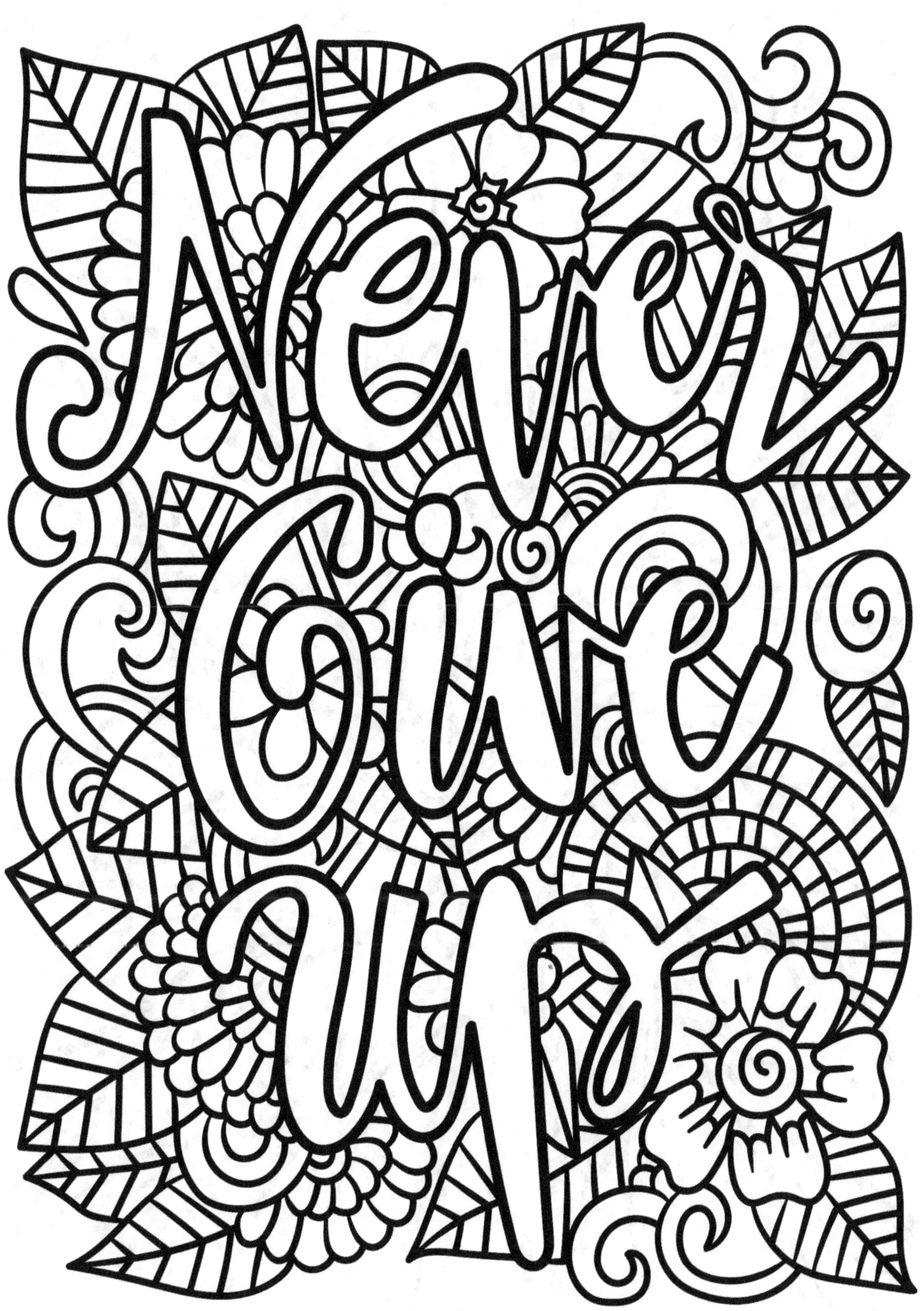

Never
Give
up

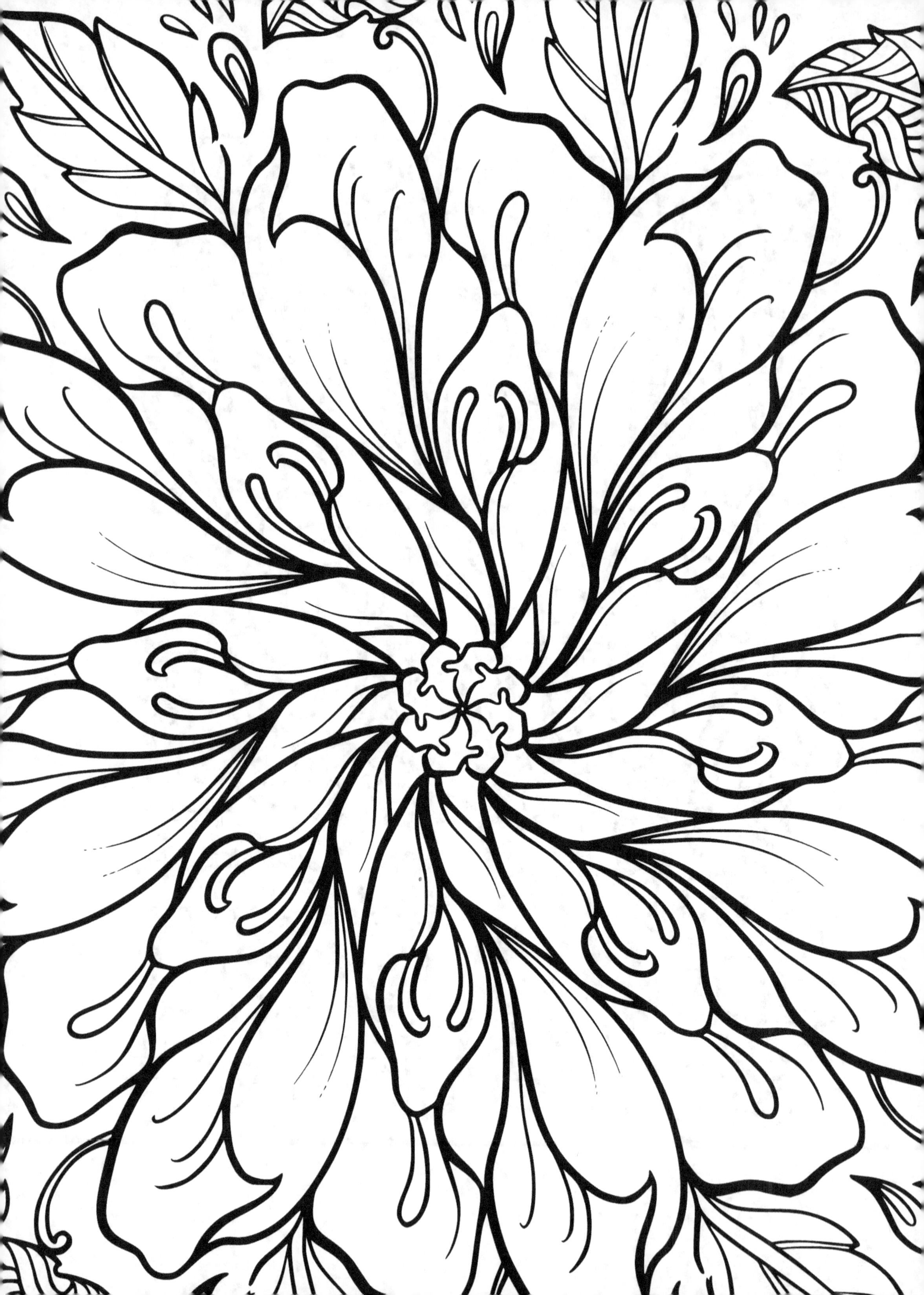

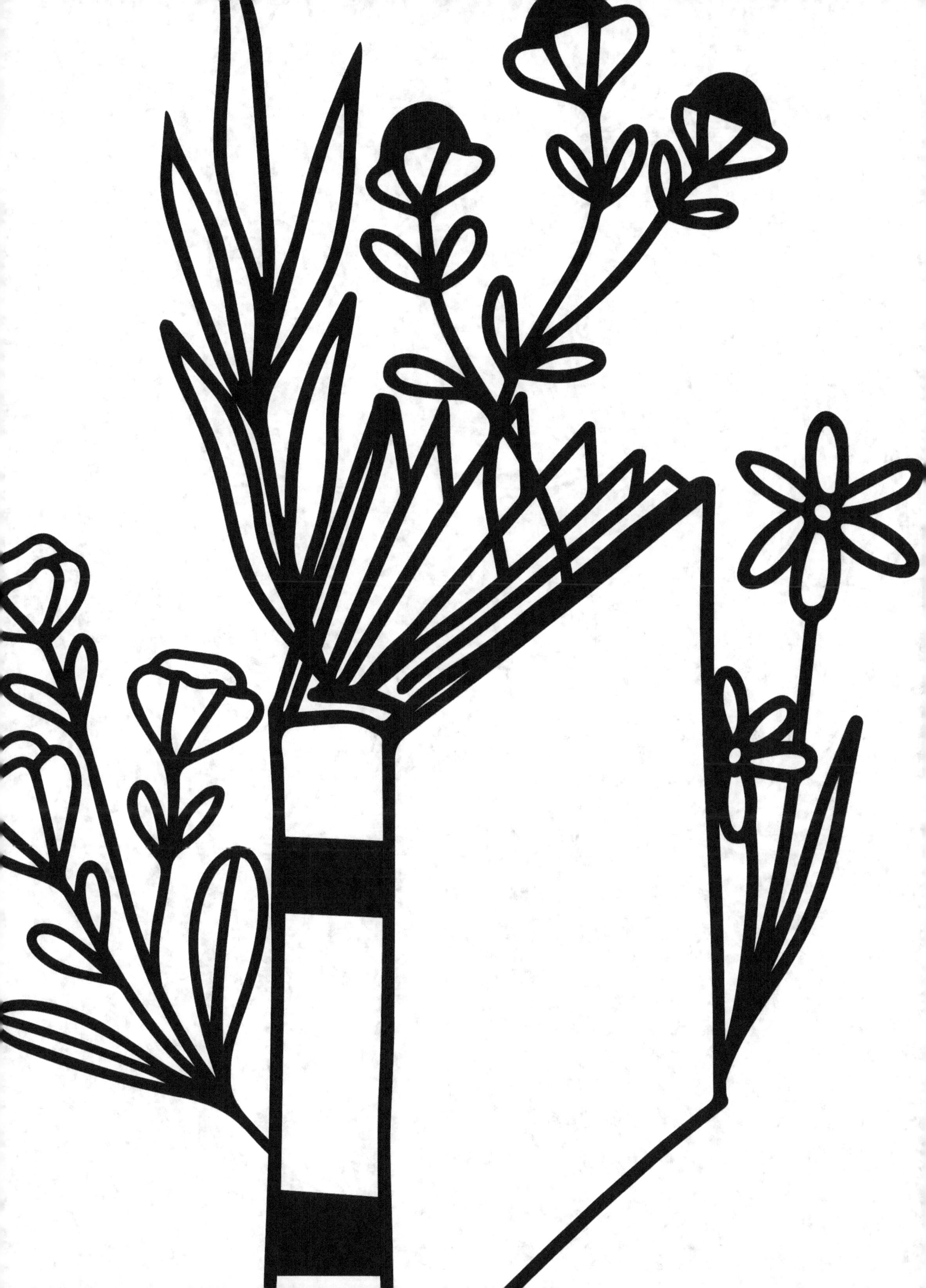

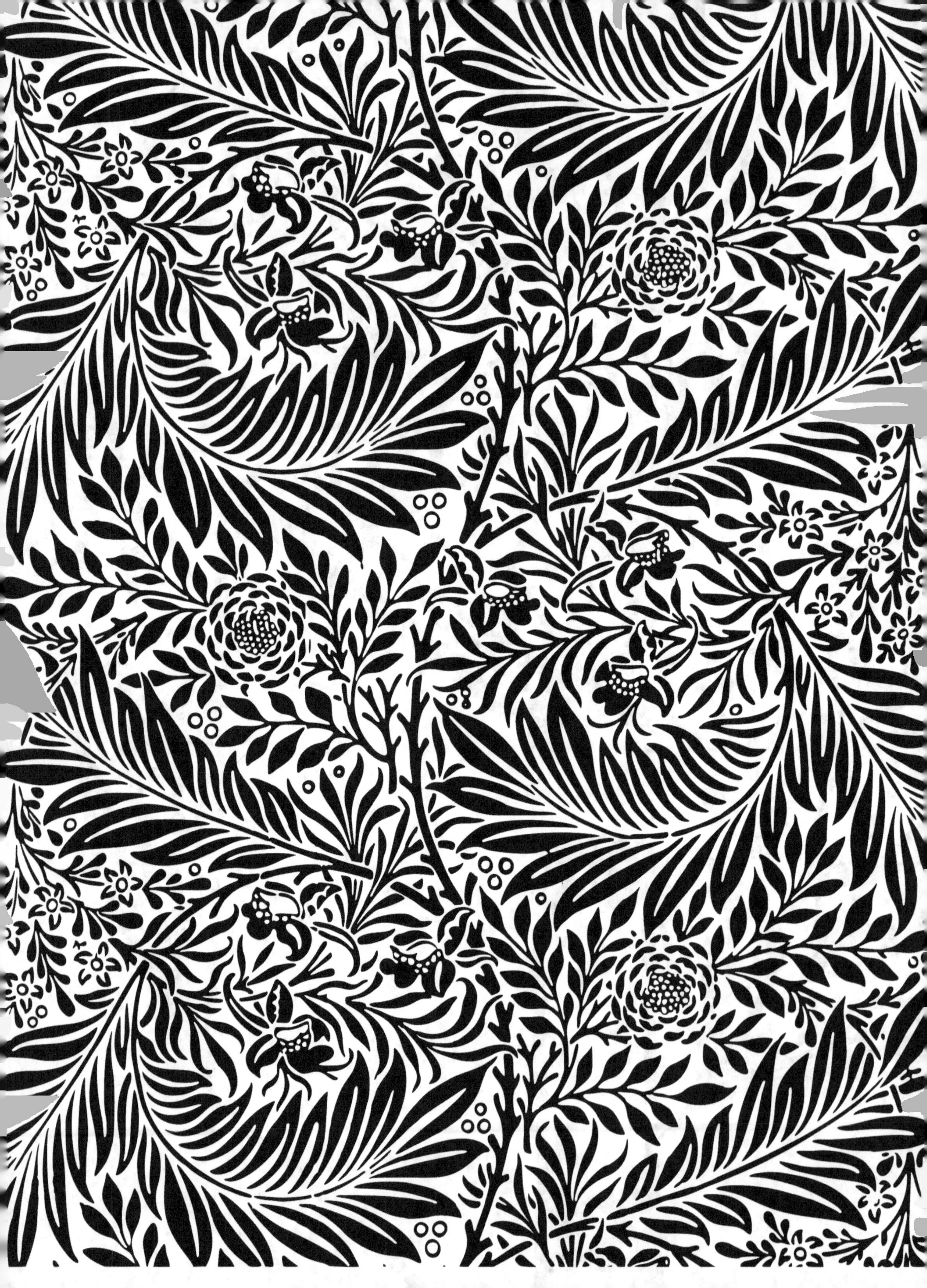

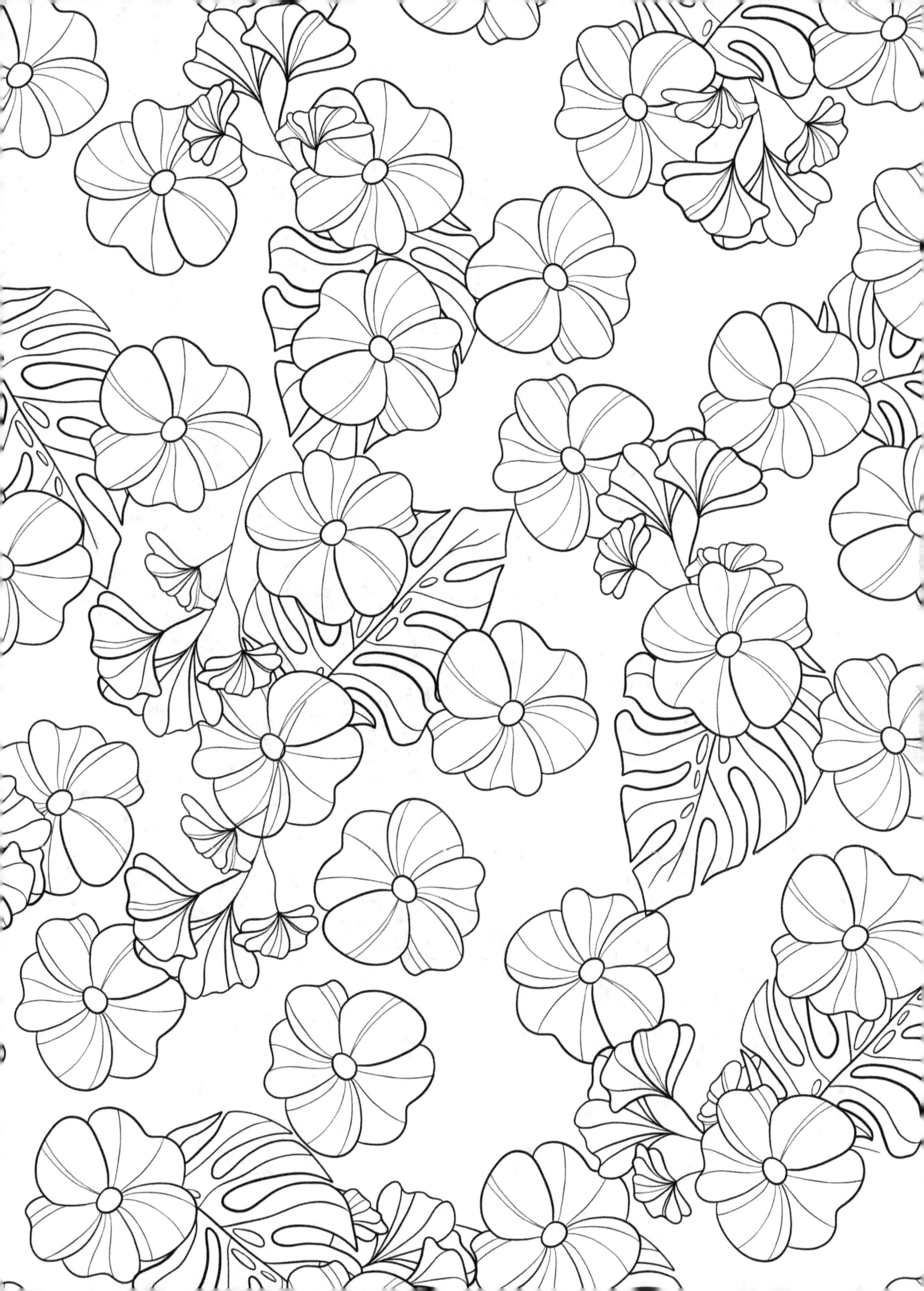

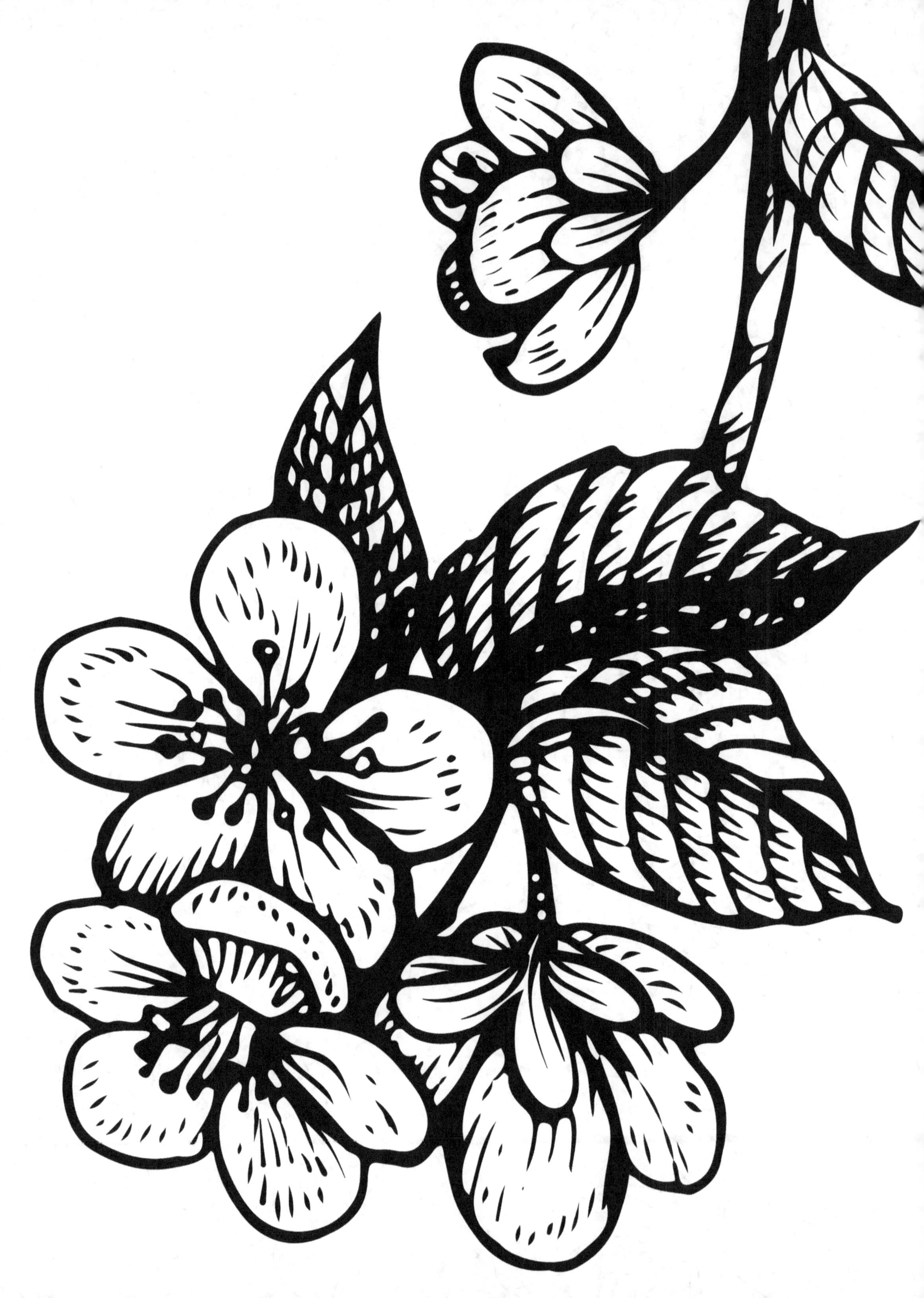

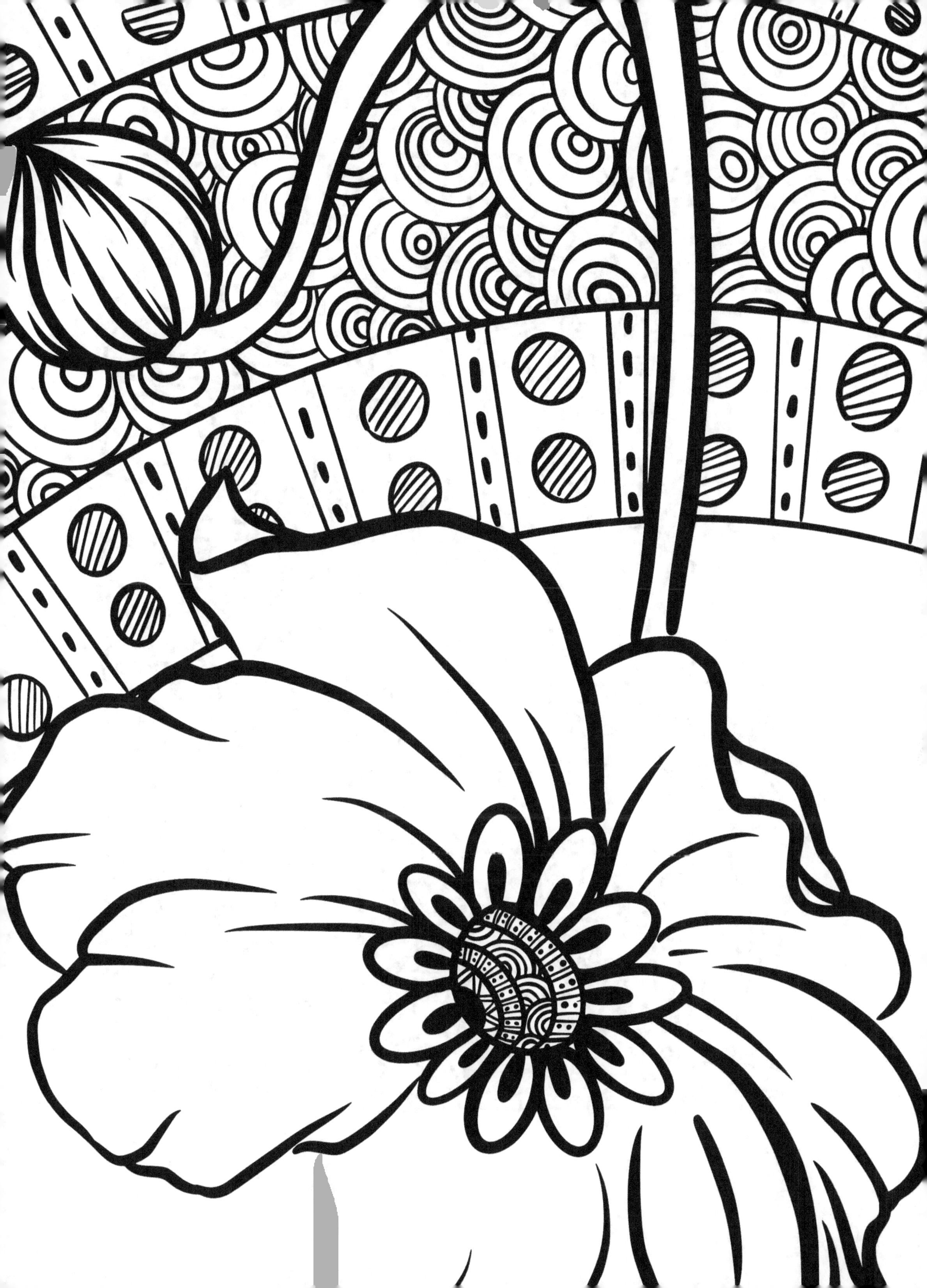

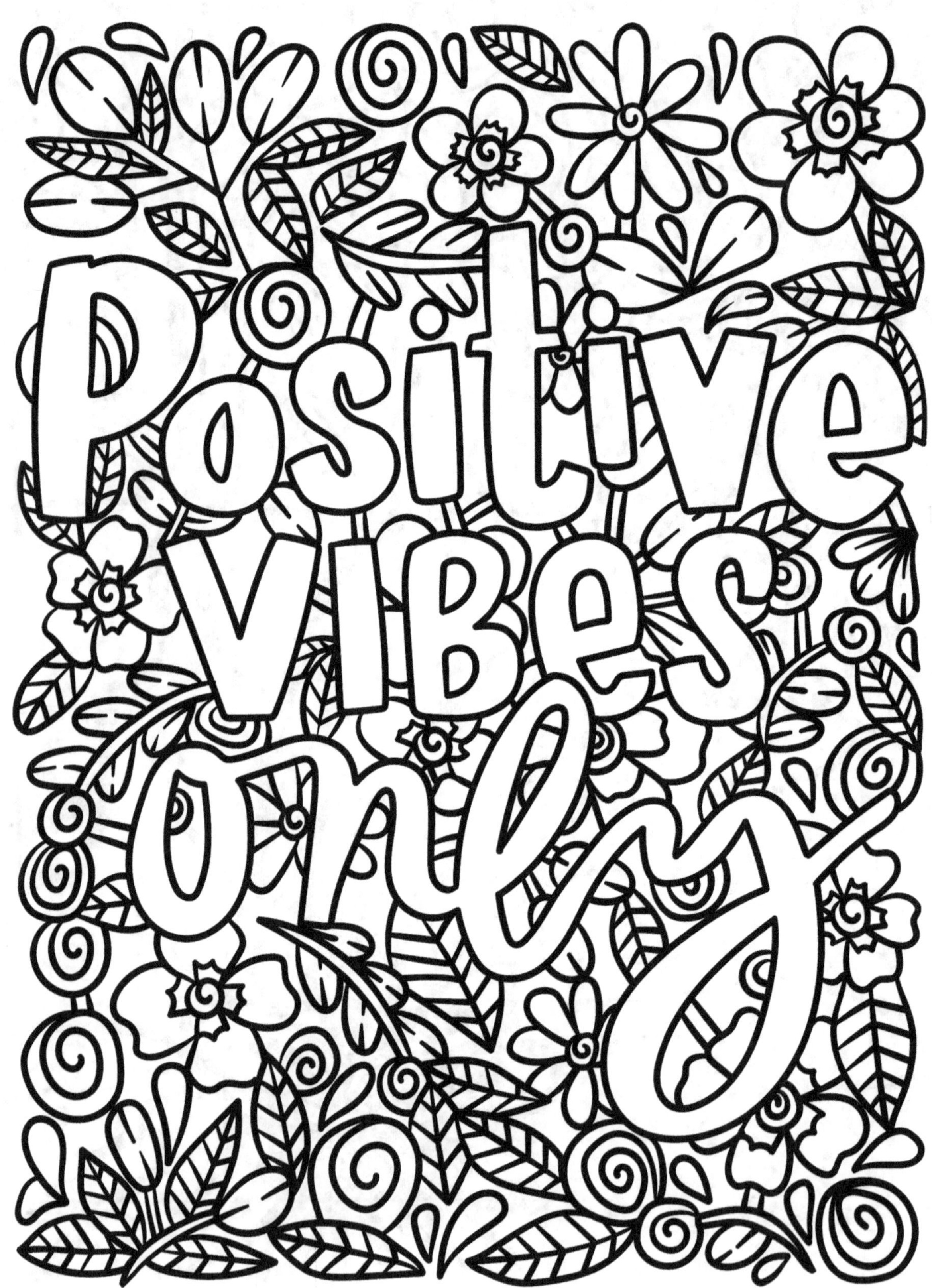

Positive
Vibes
only

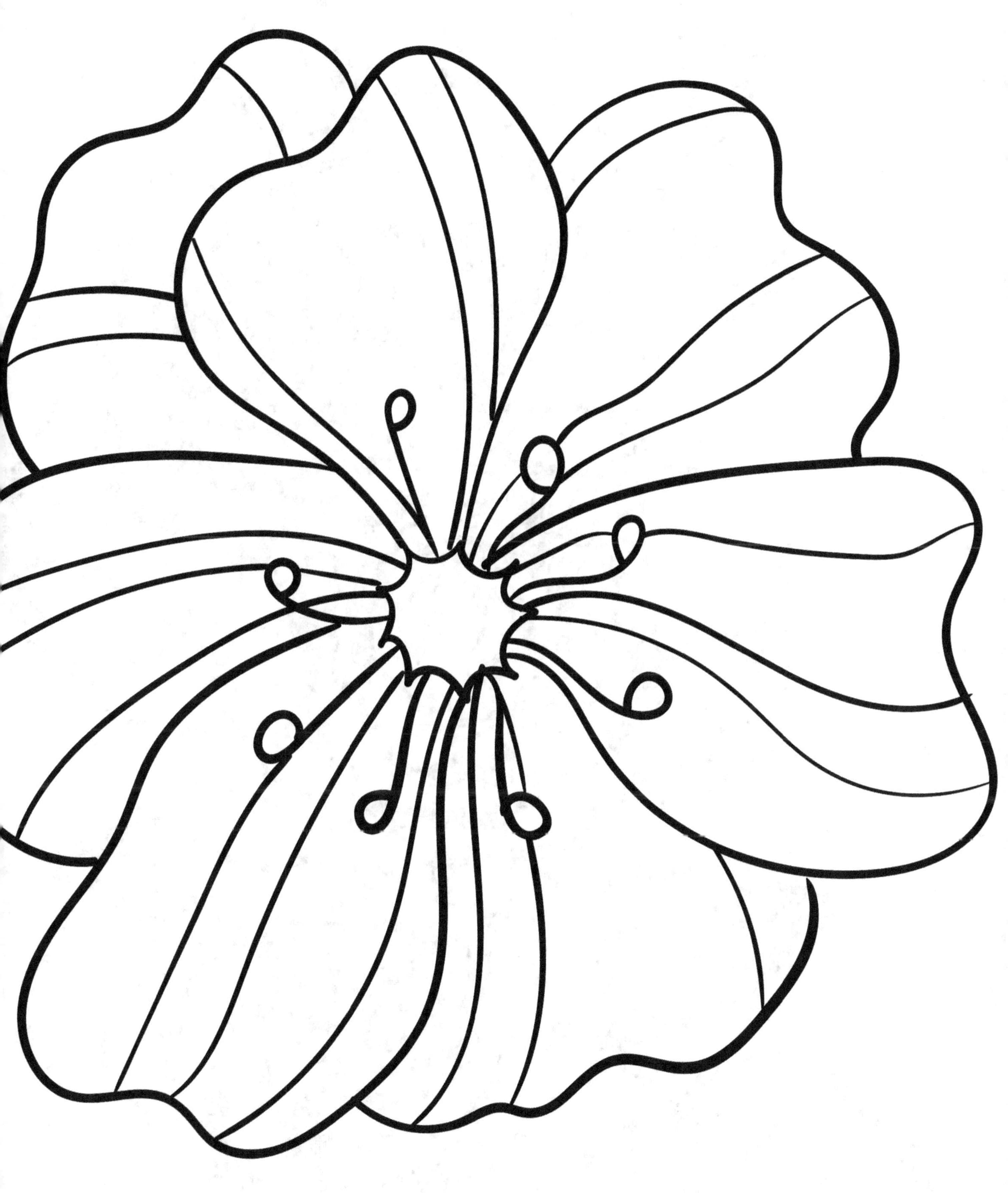

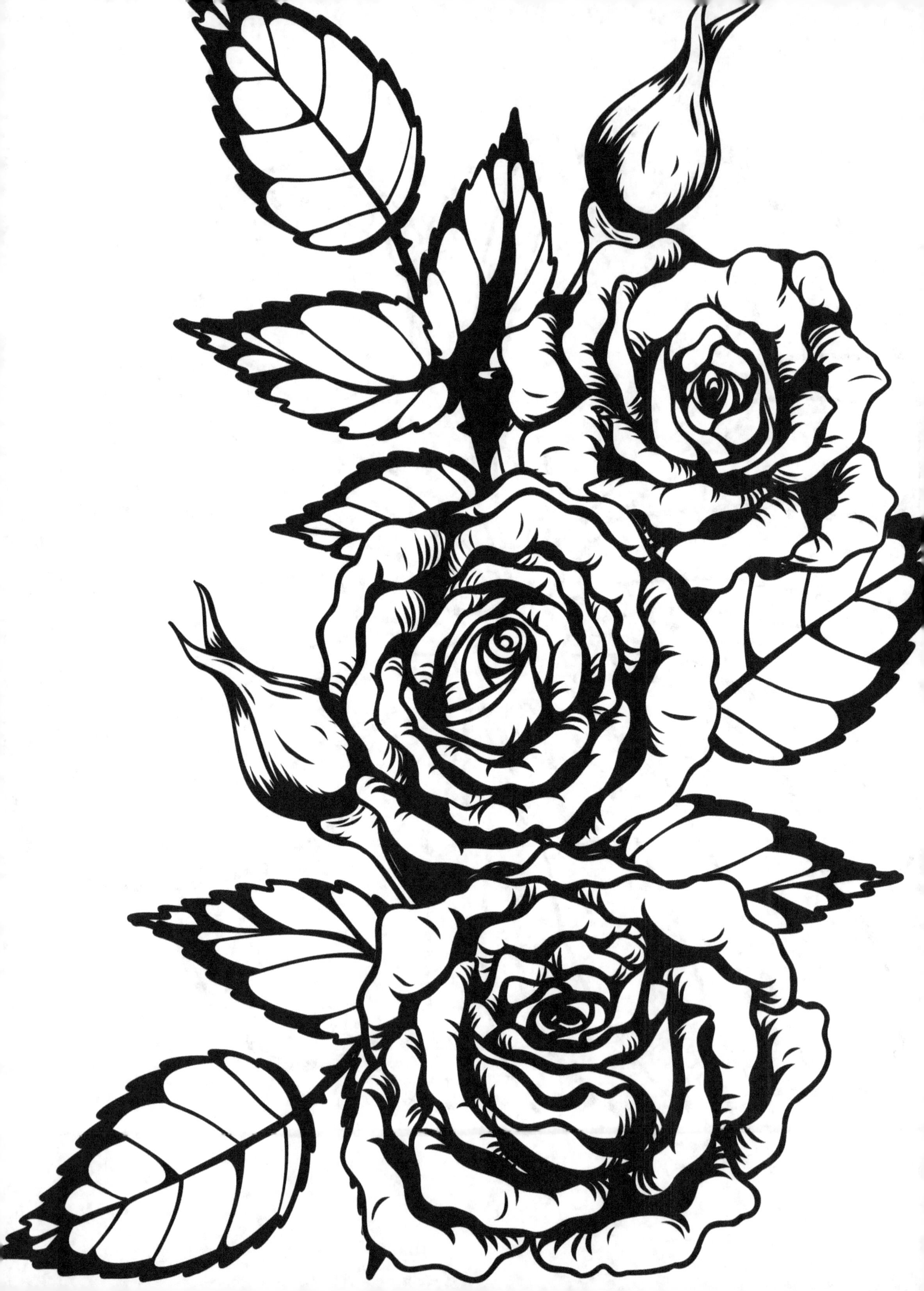

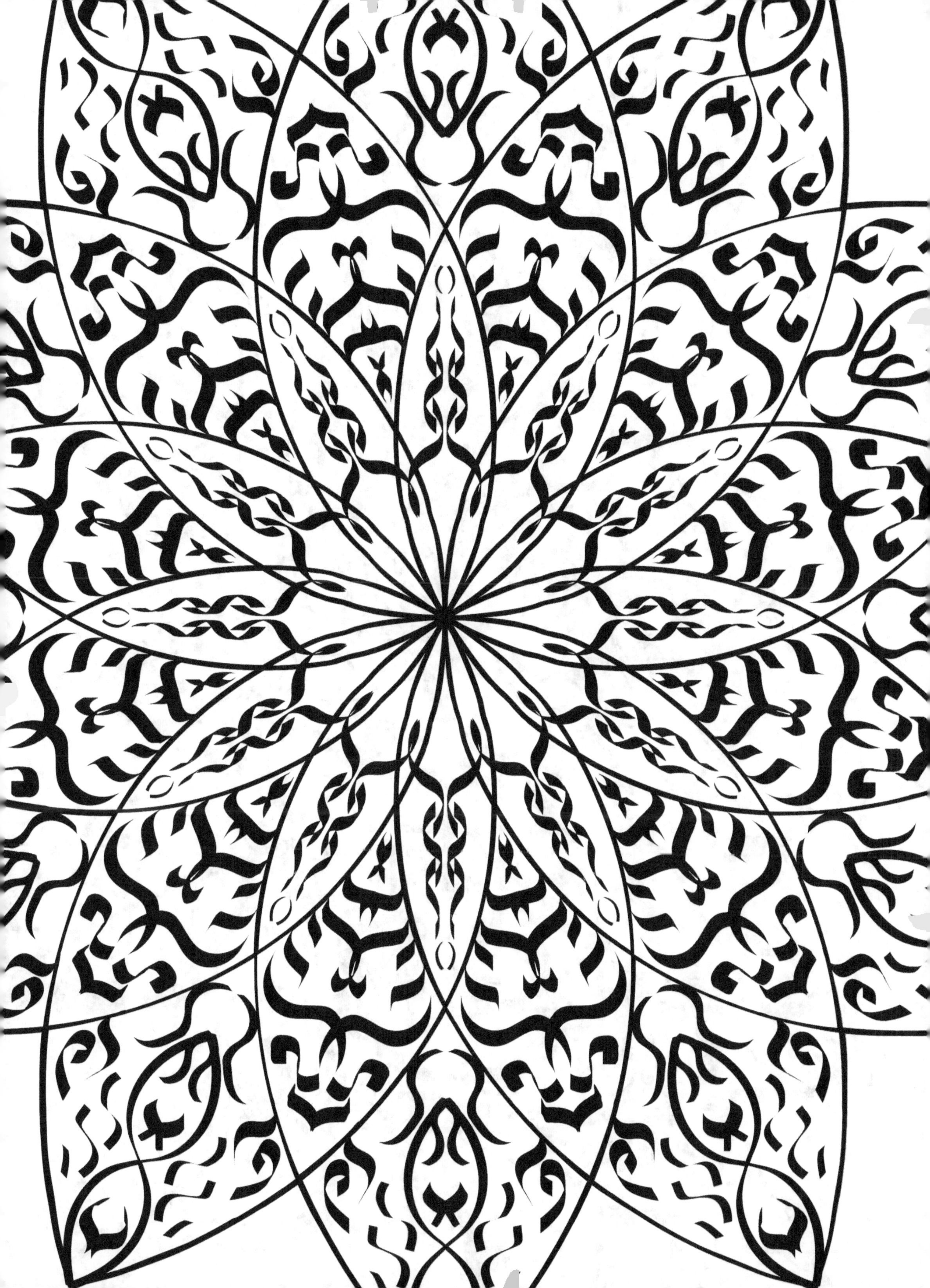

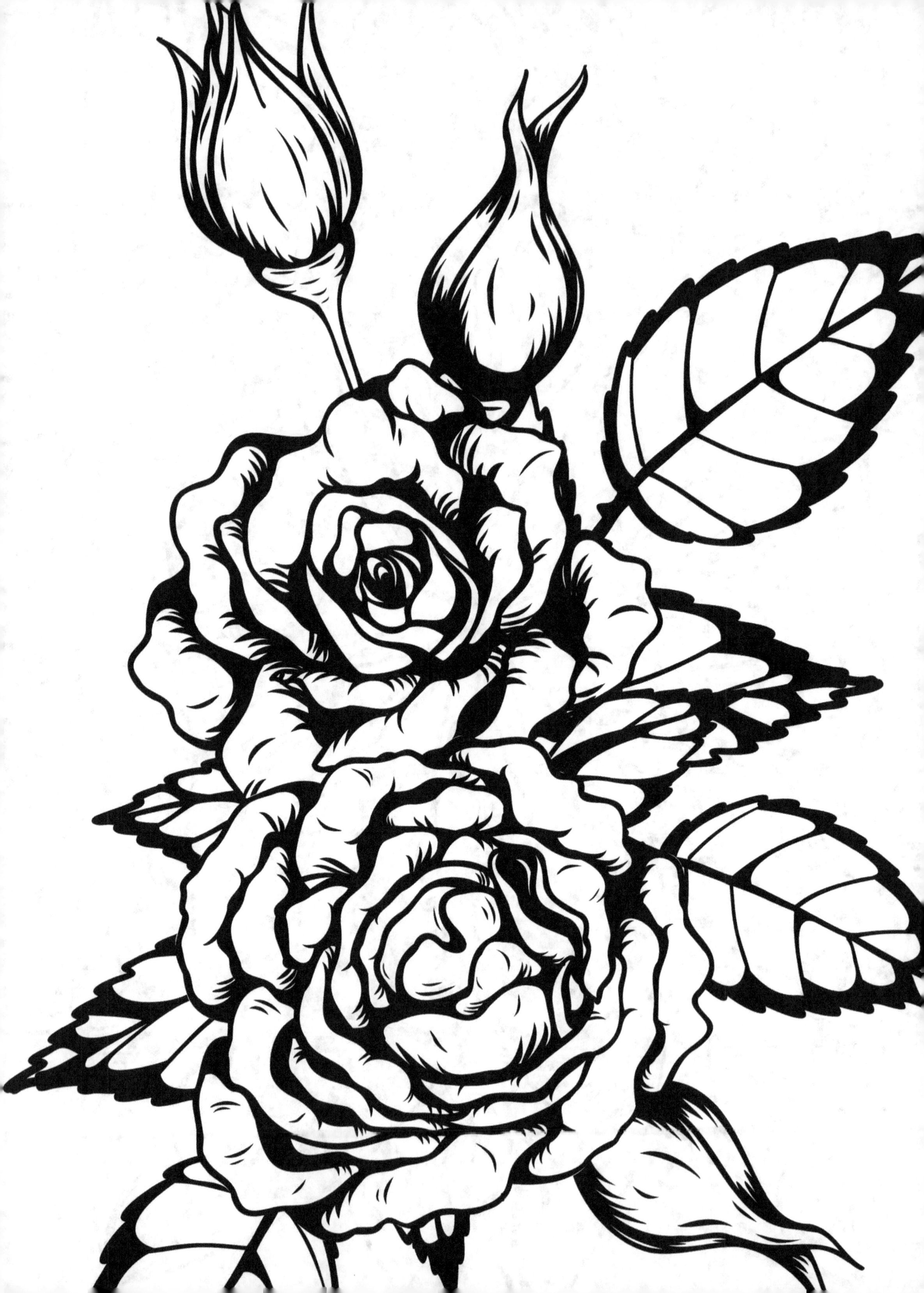

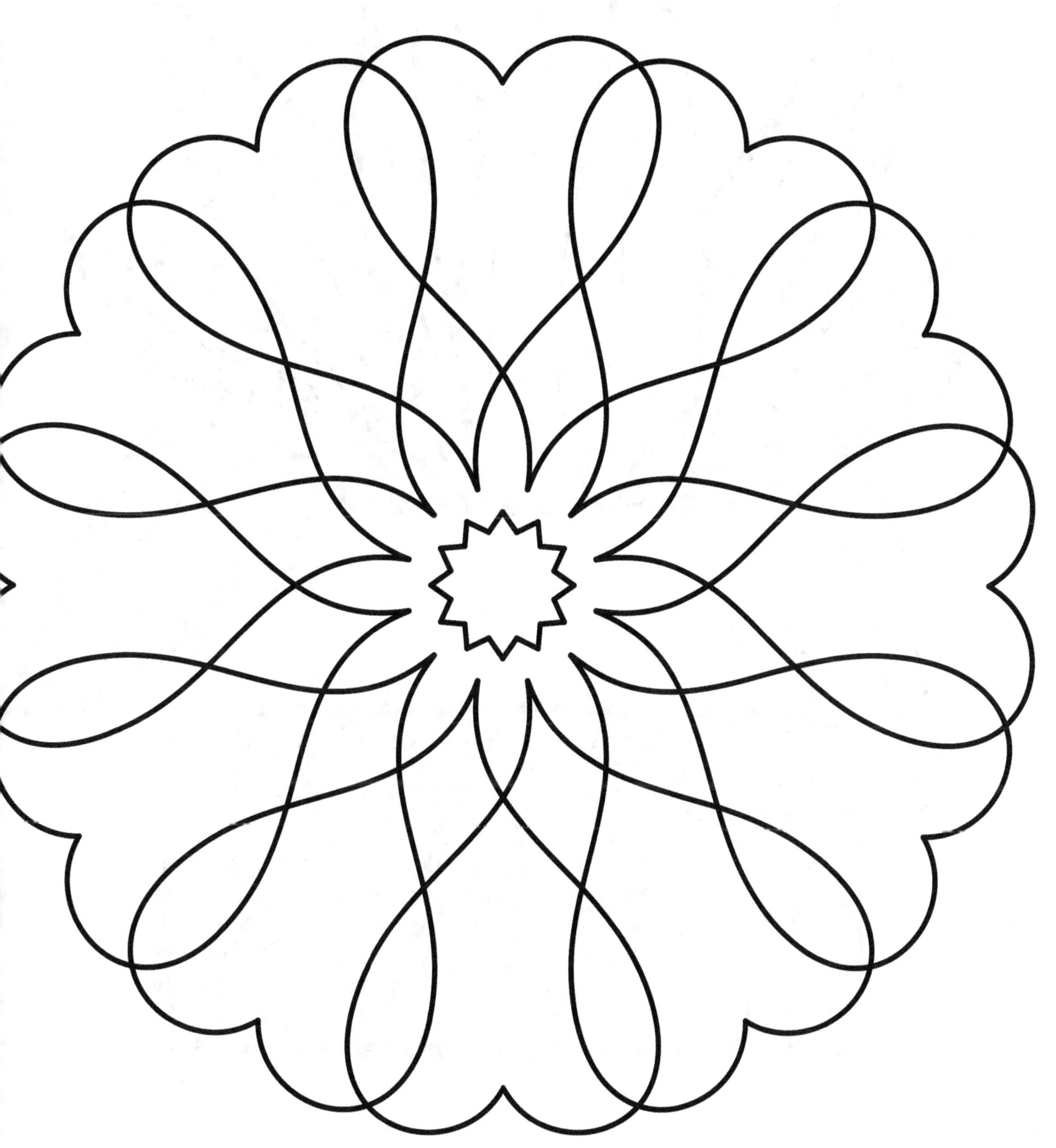

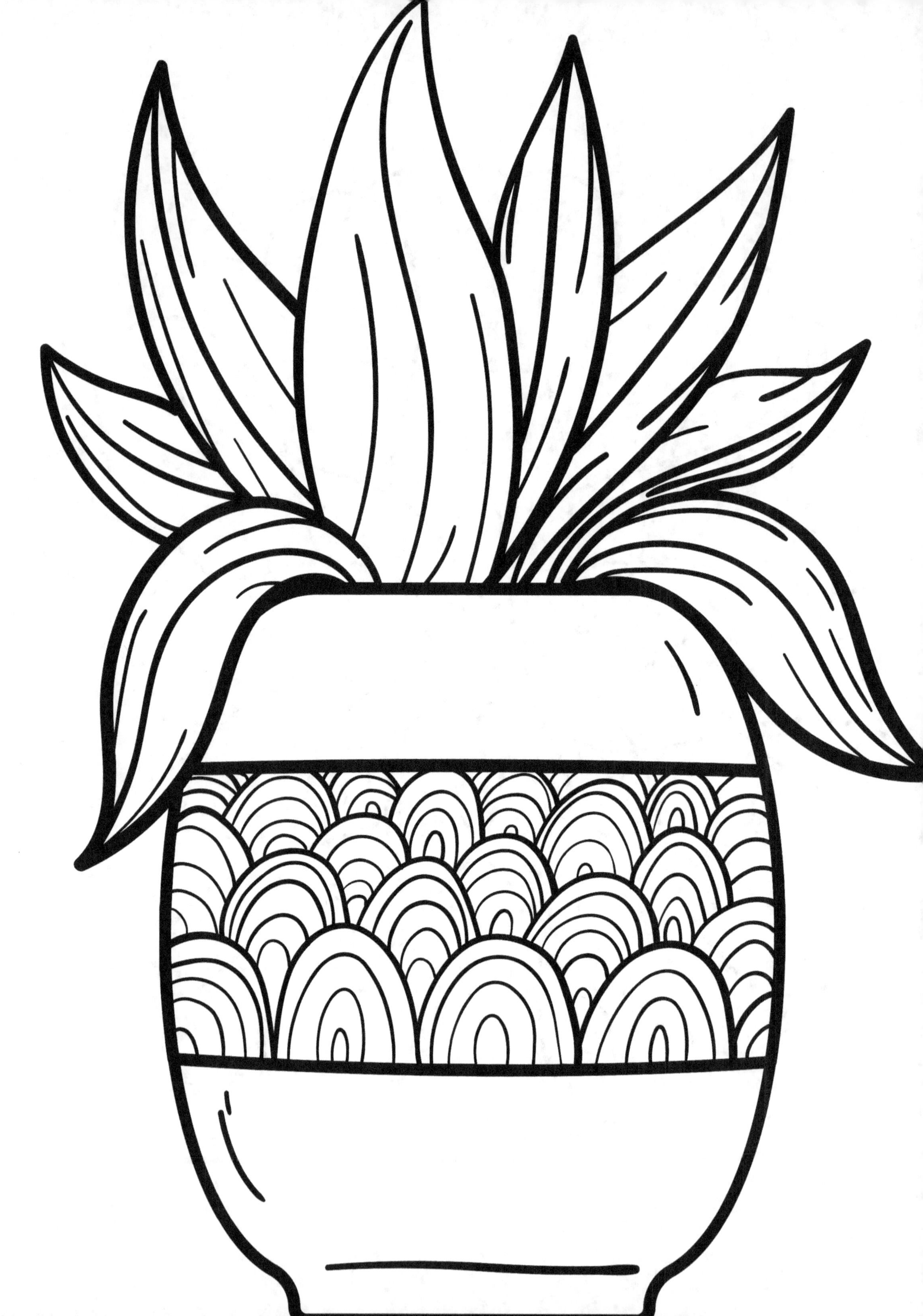

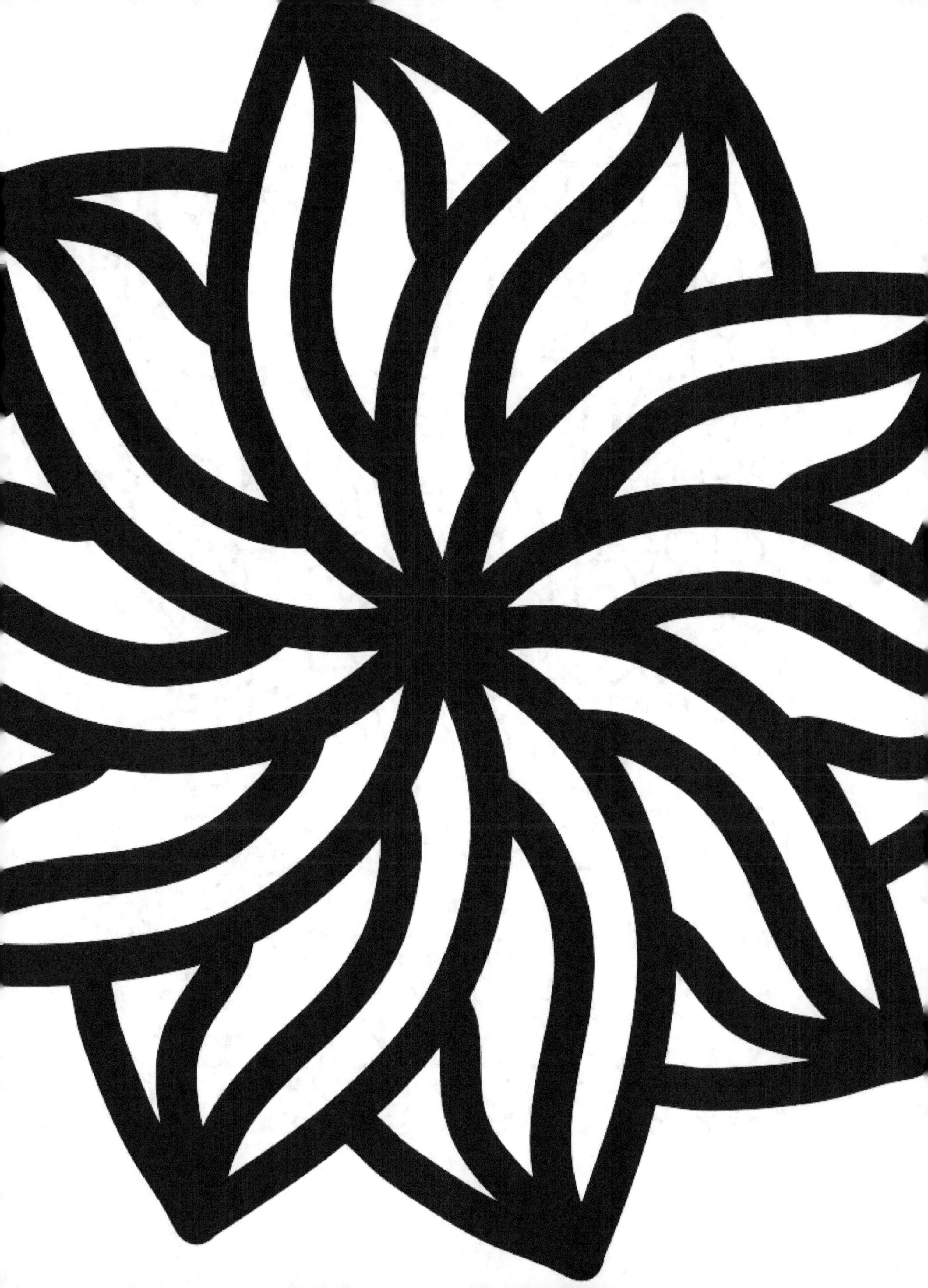

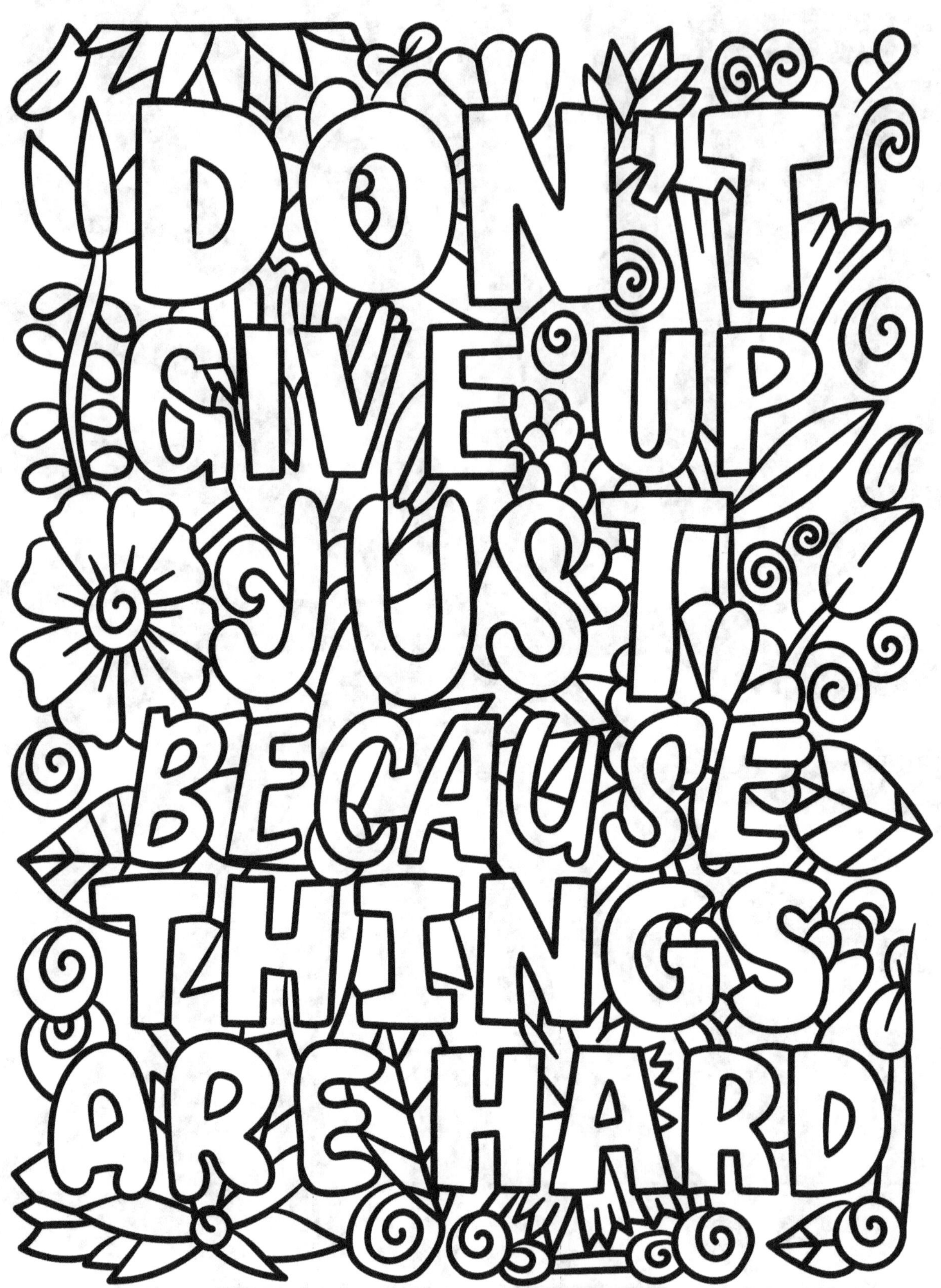

Don't
Give Up
Just
Because
Things
Are Hard

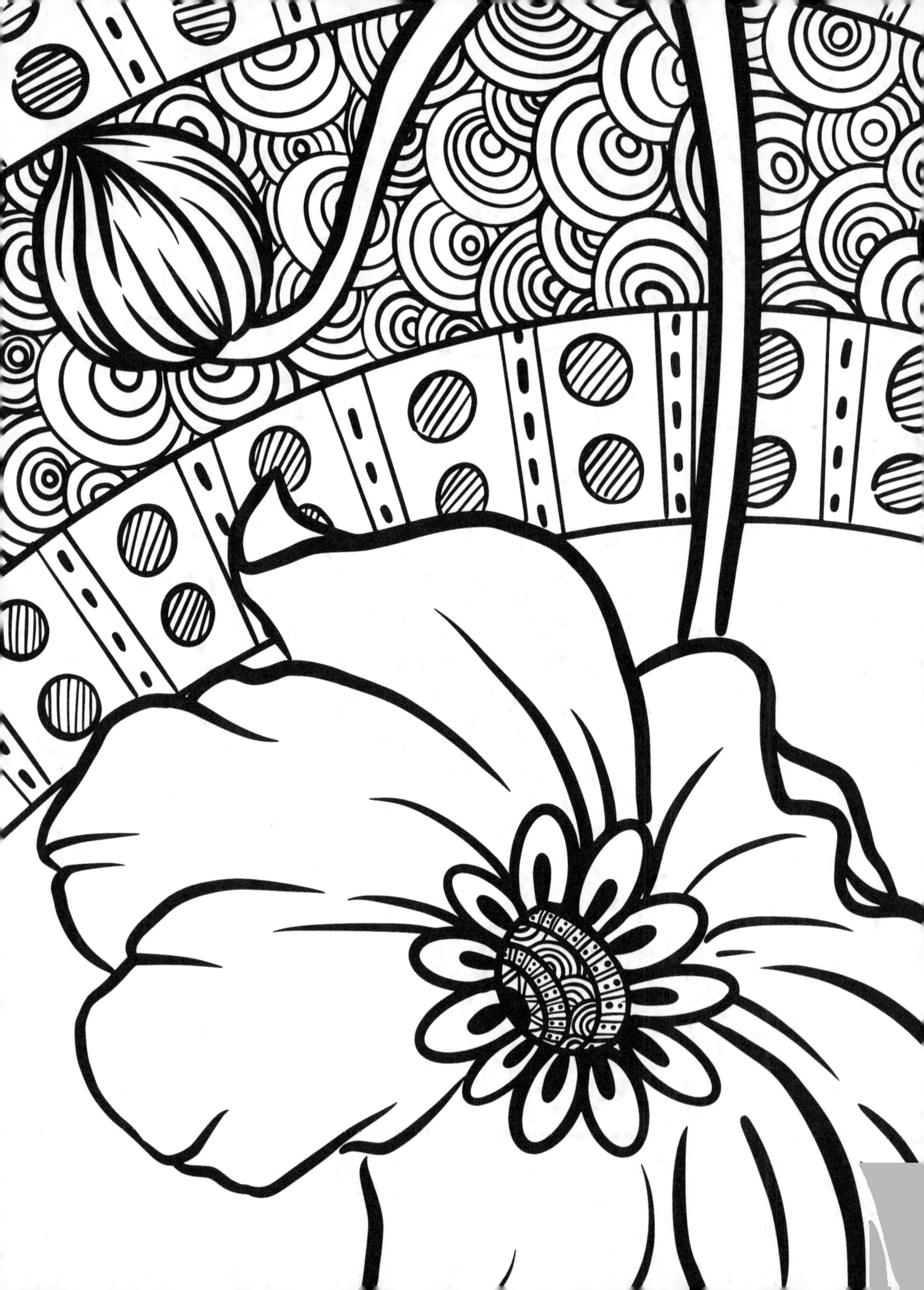

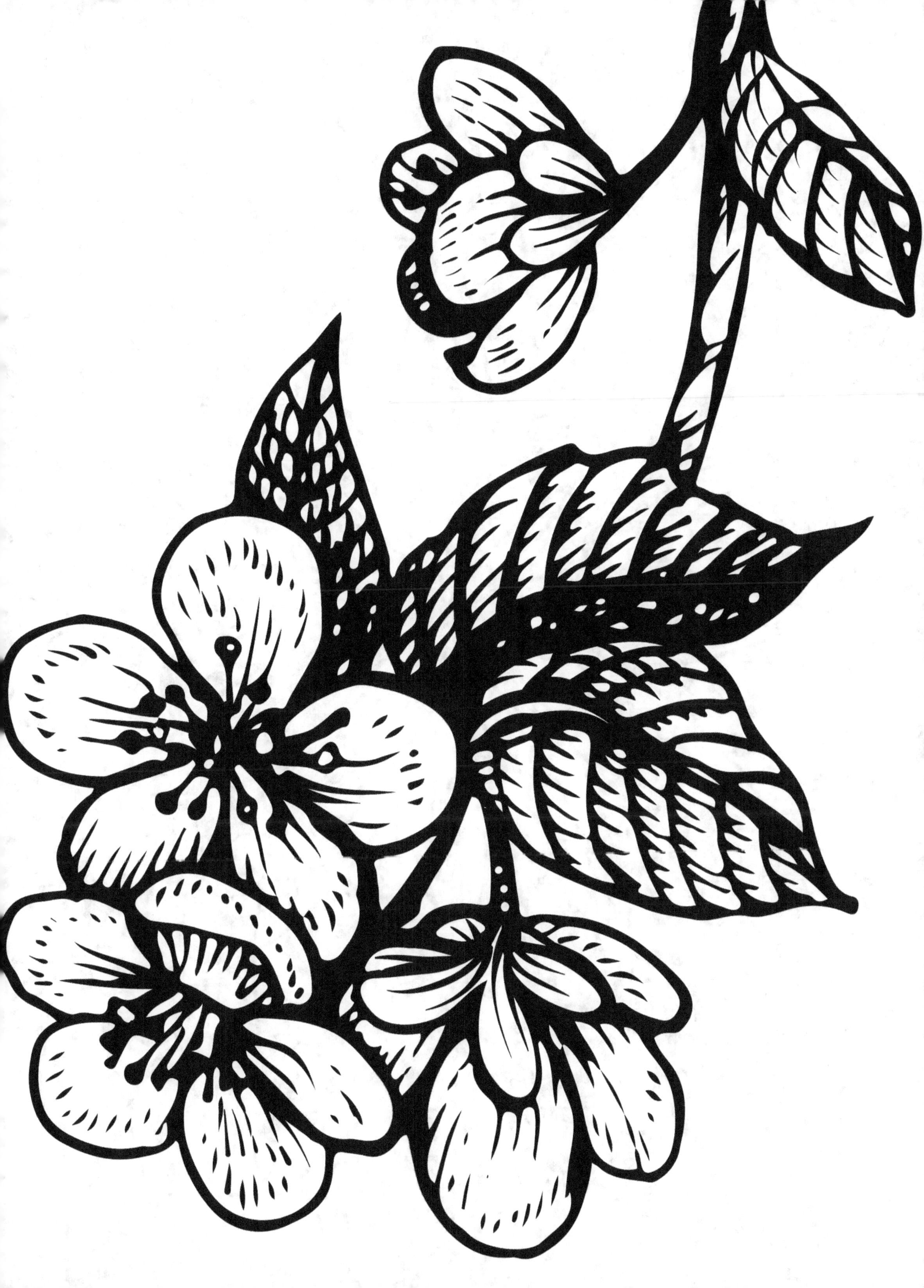

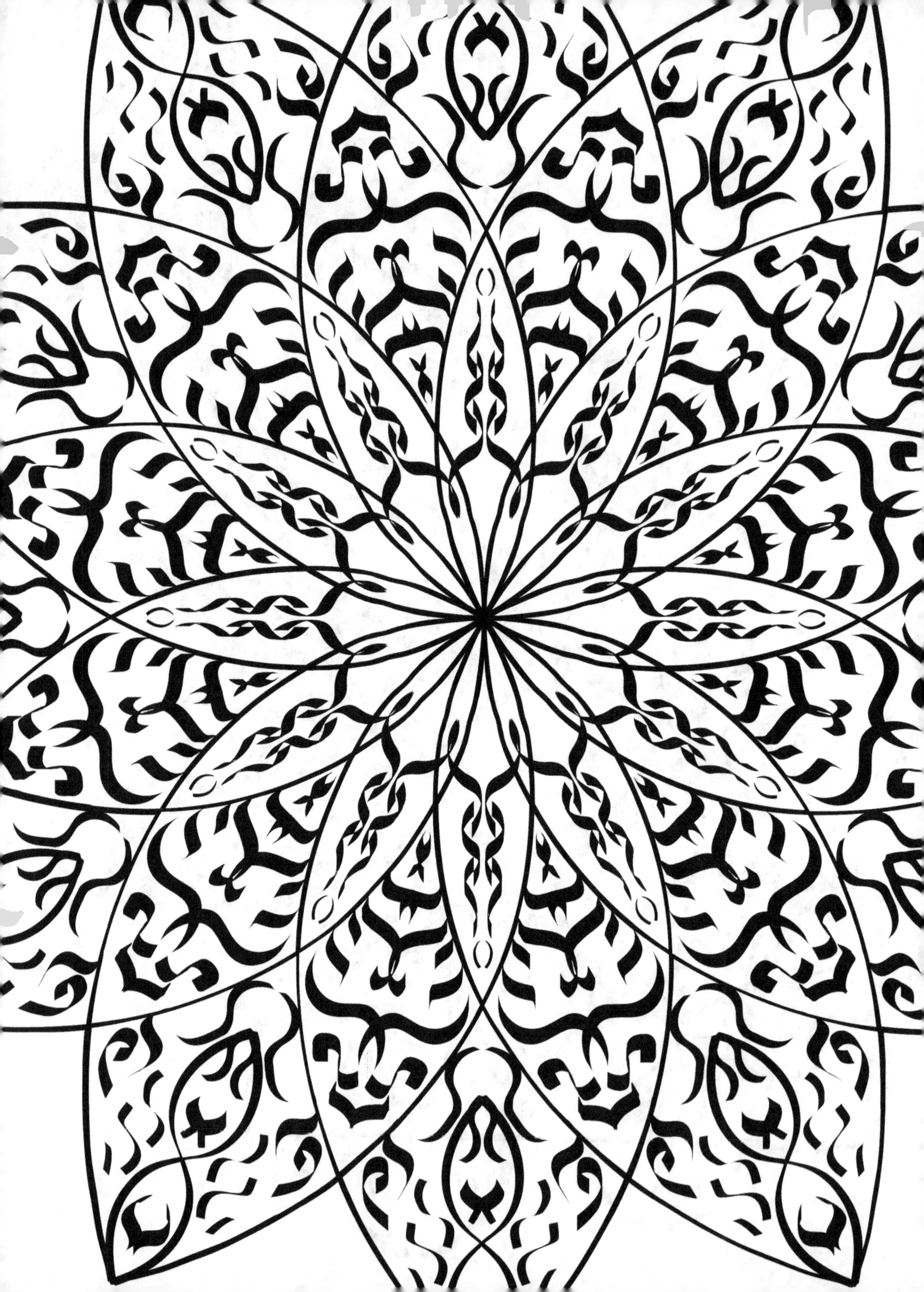

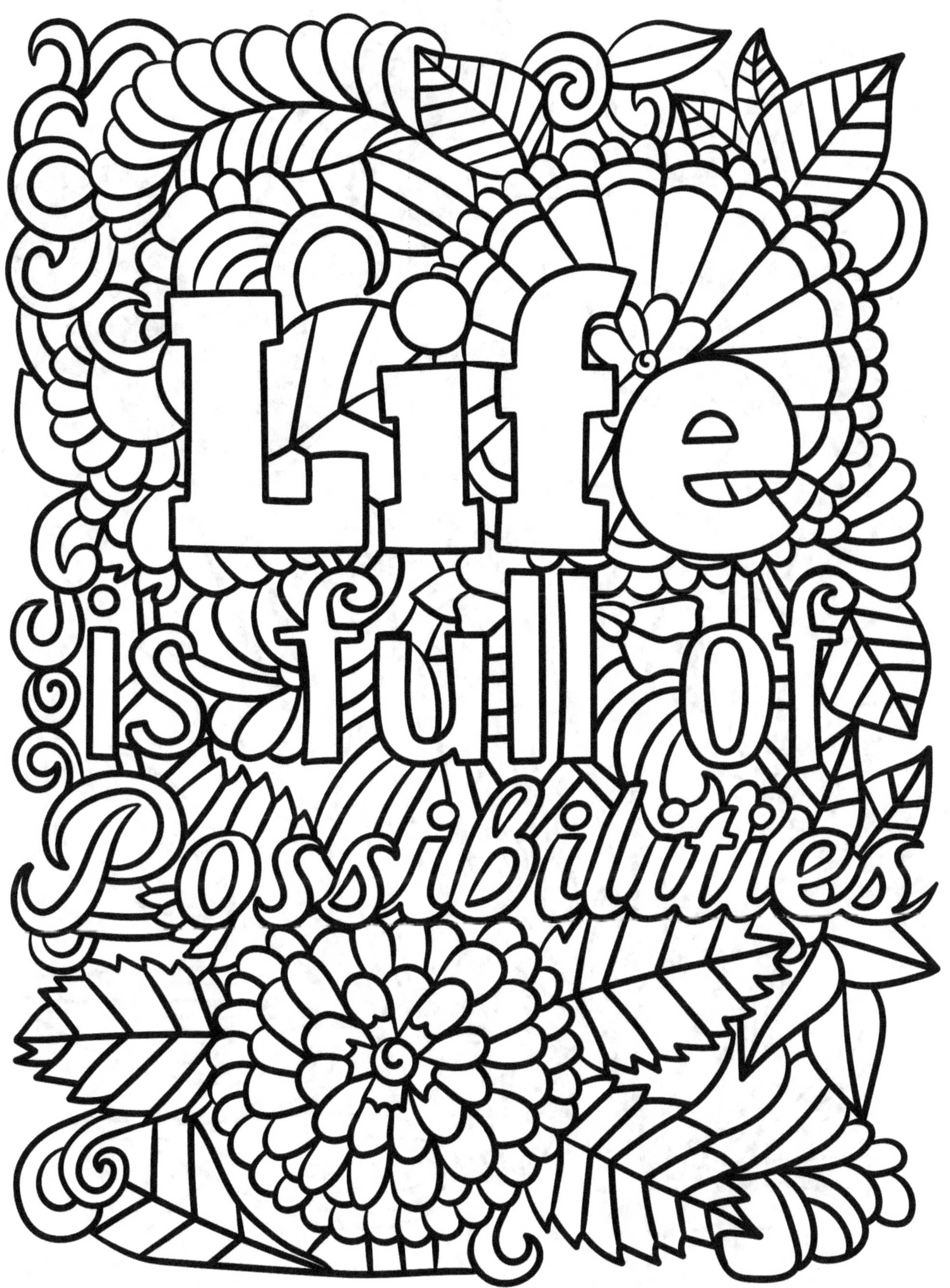

Life
is full of
Possibilities

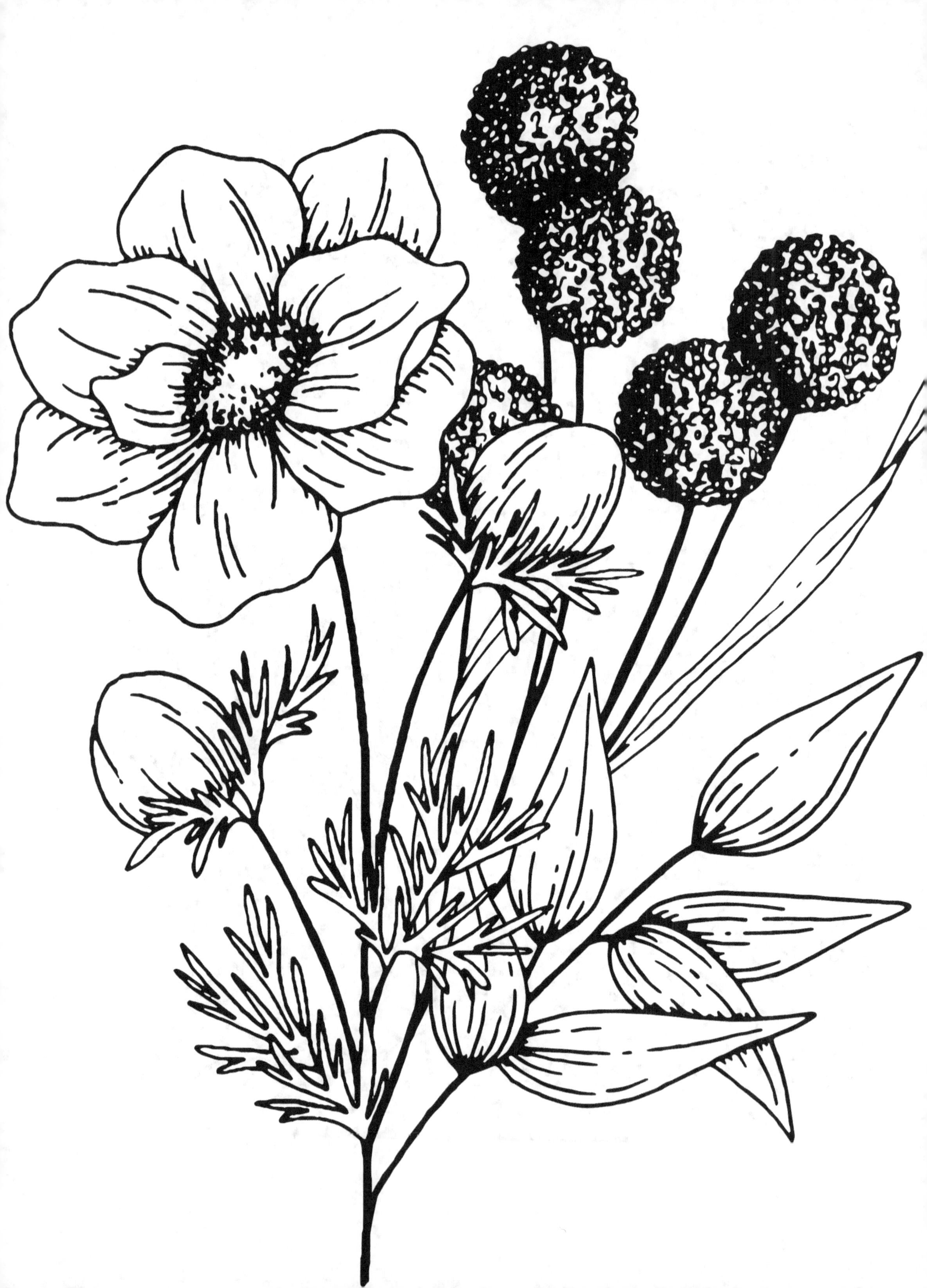

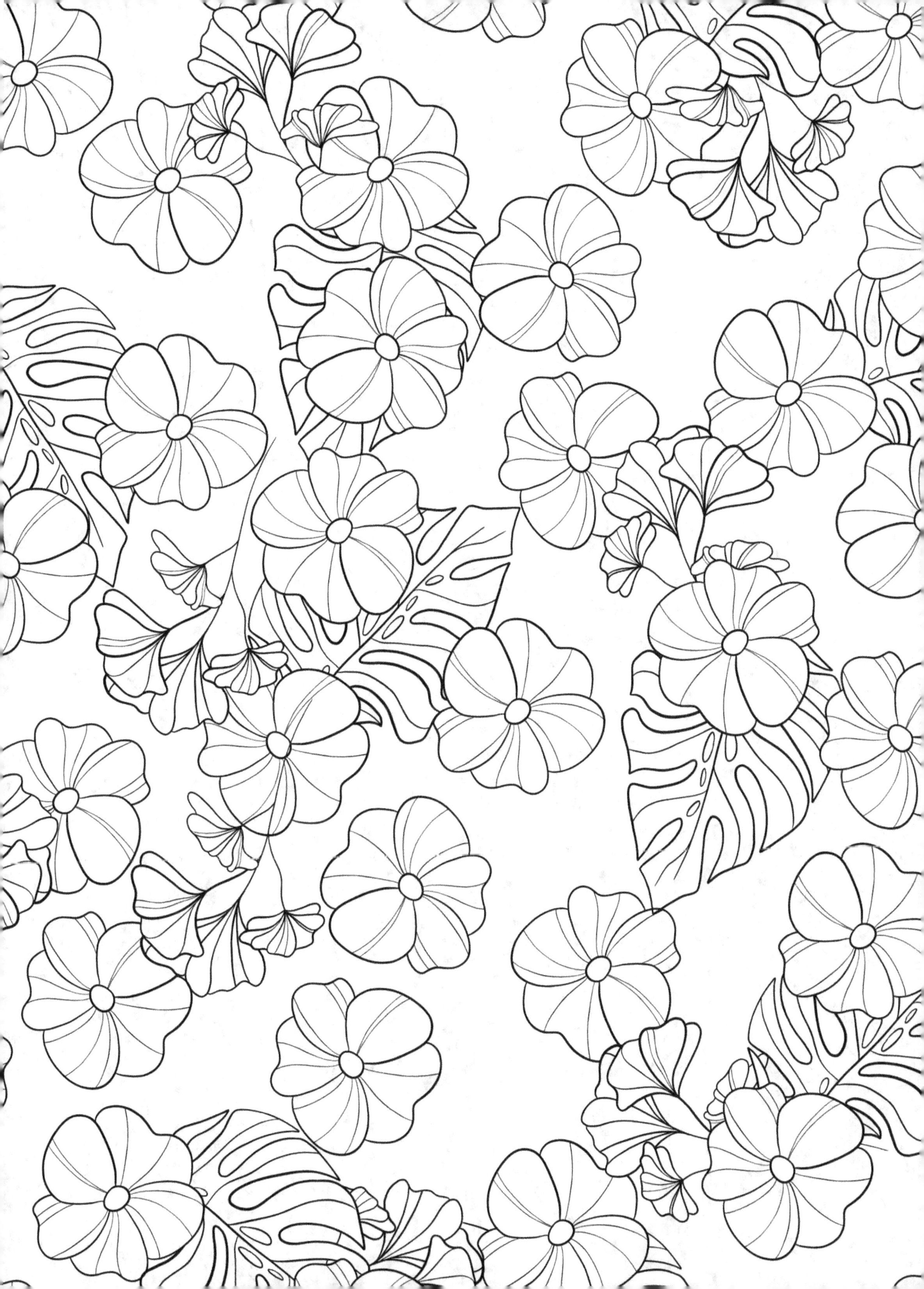

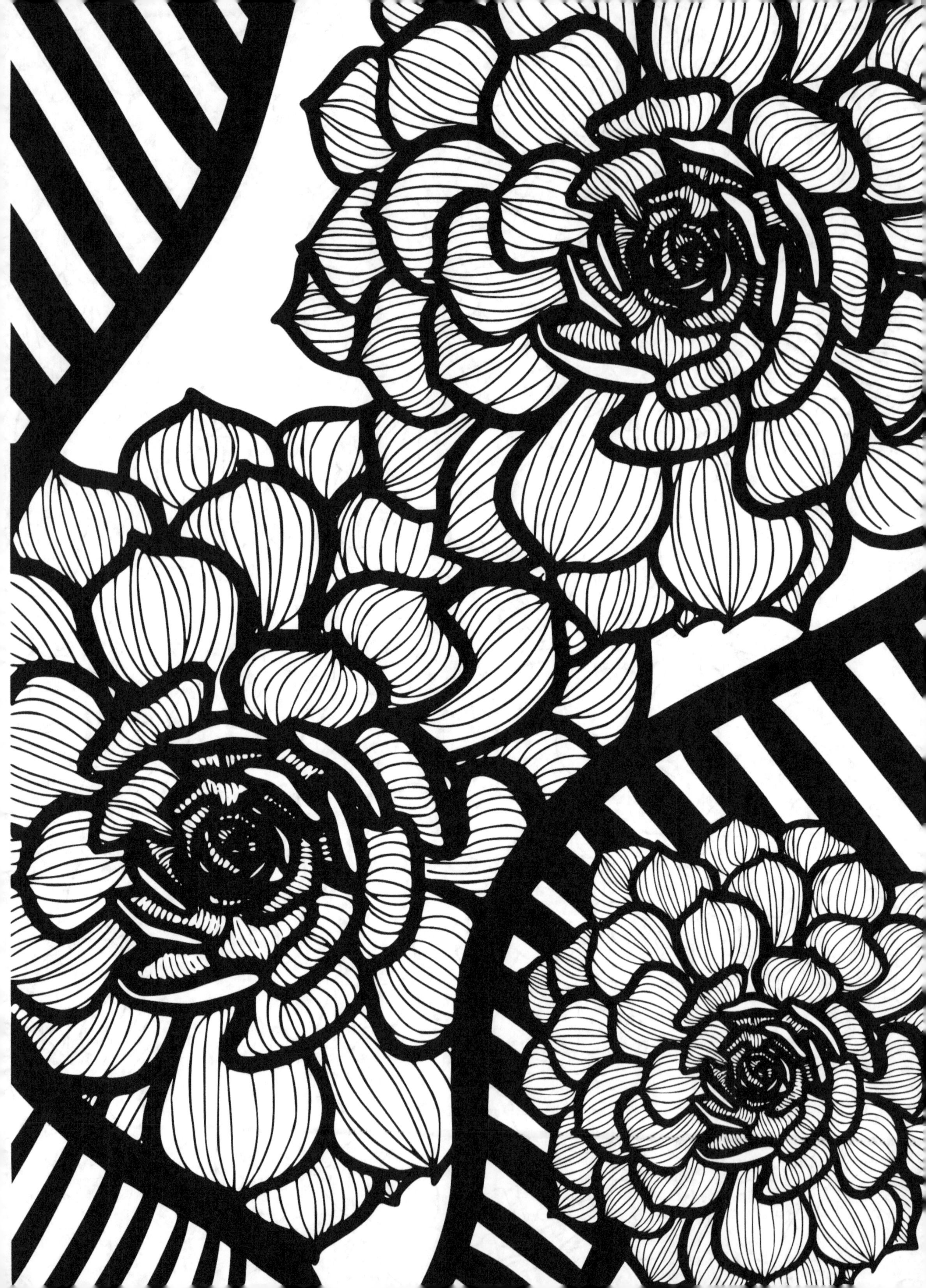

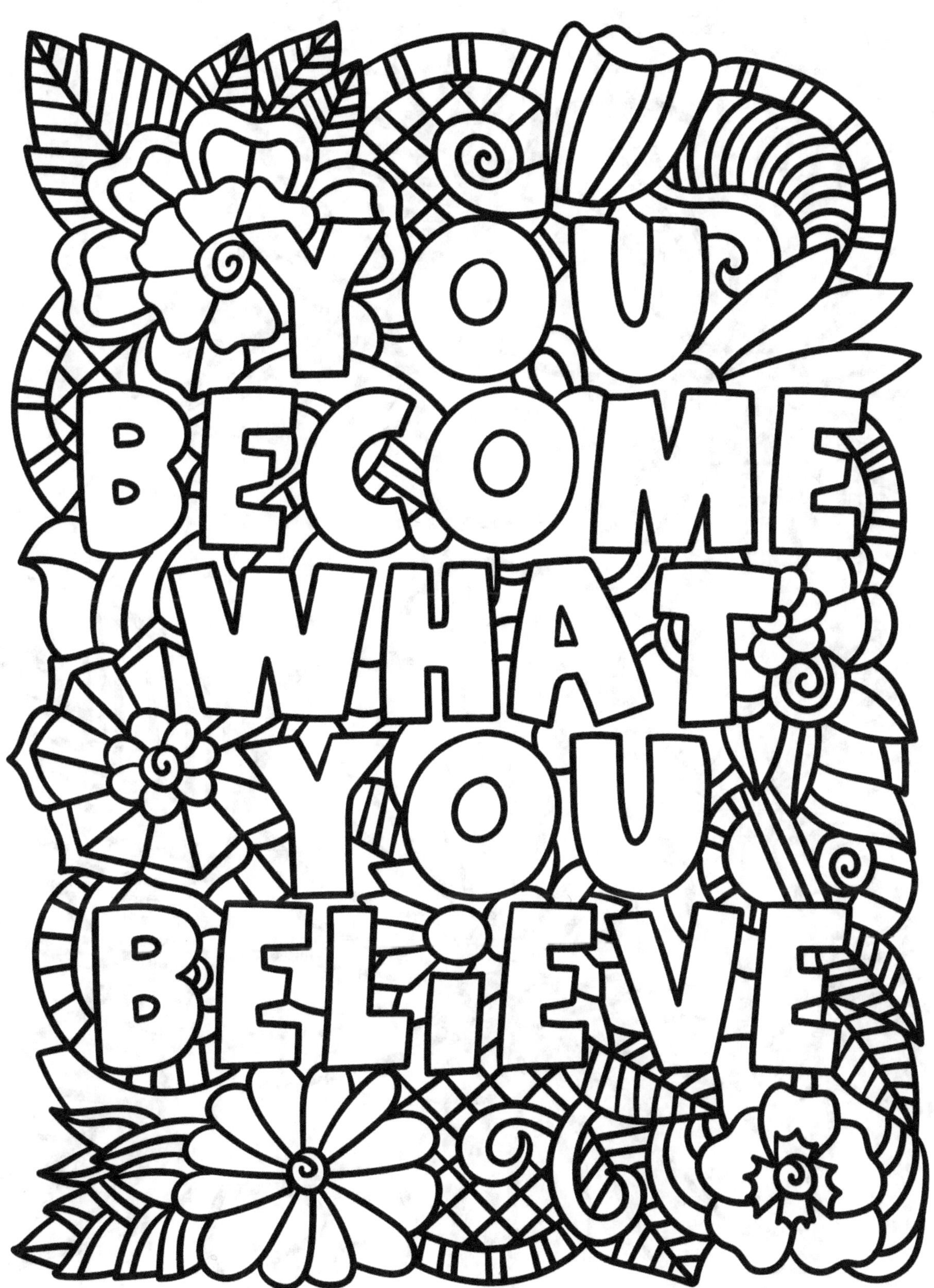

YOU
BECOME
WHAT
YOU
BELIEVE

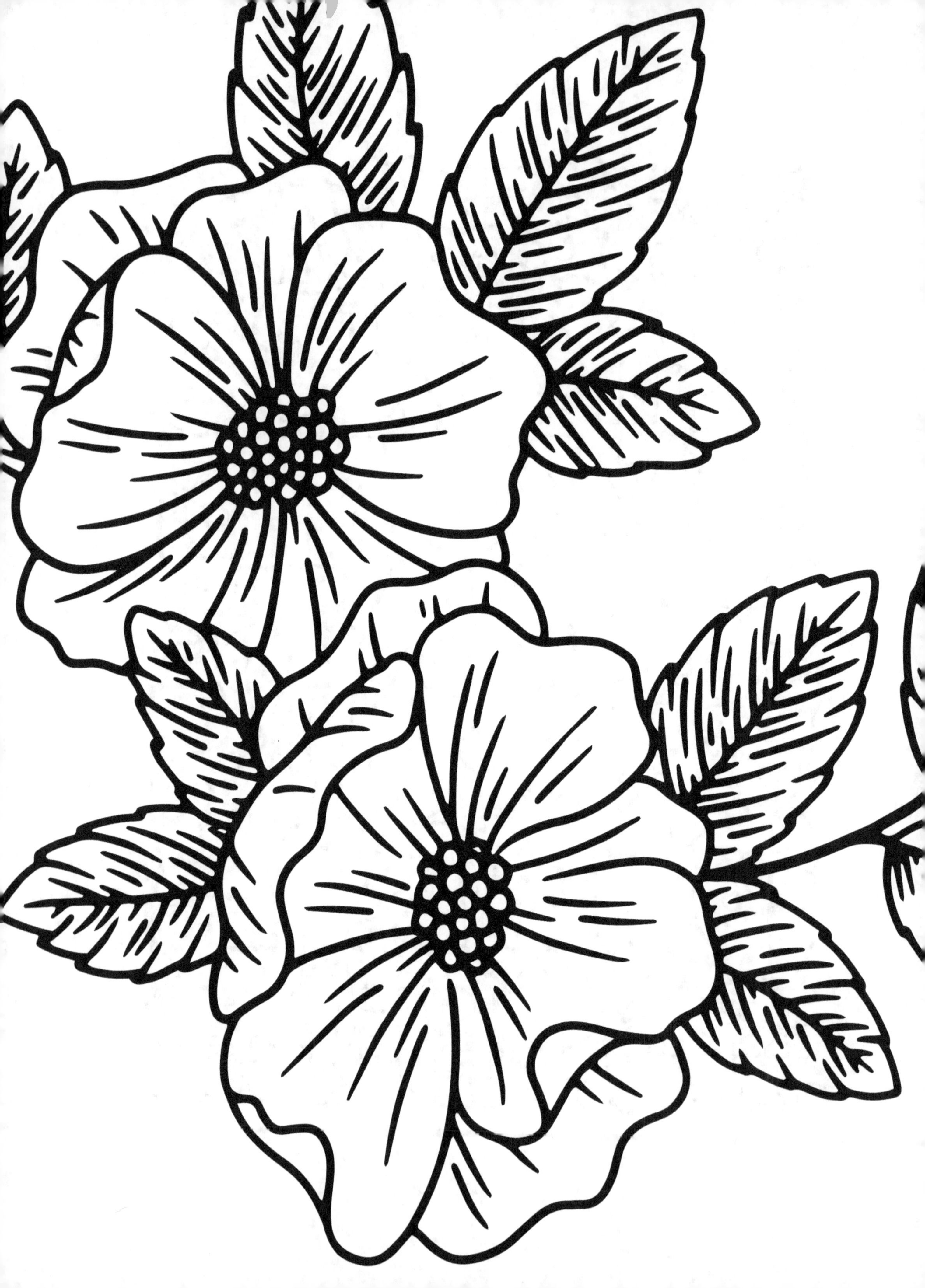

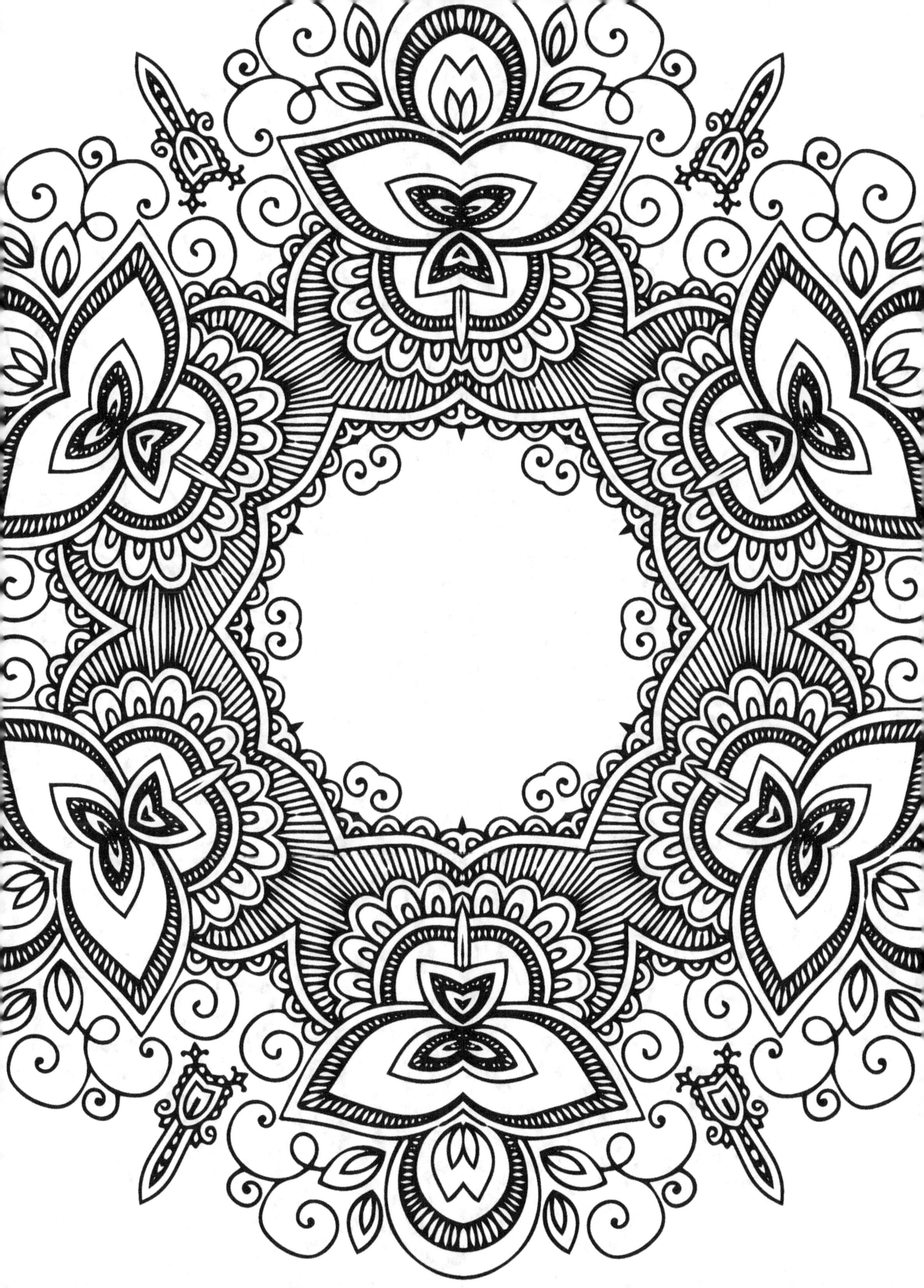

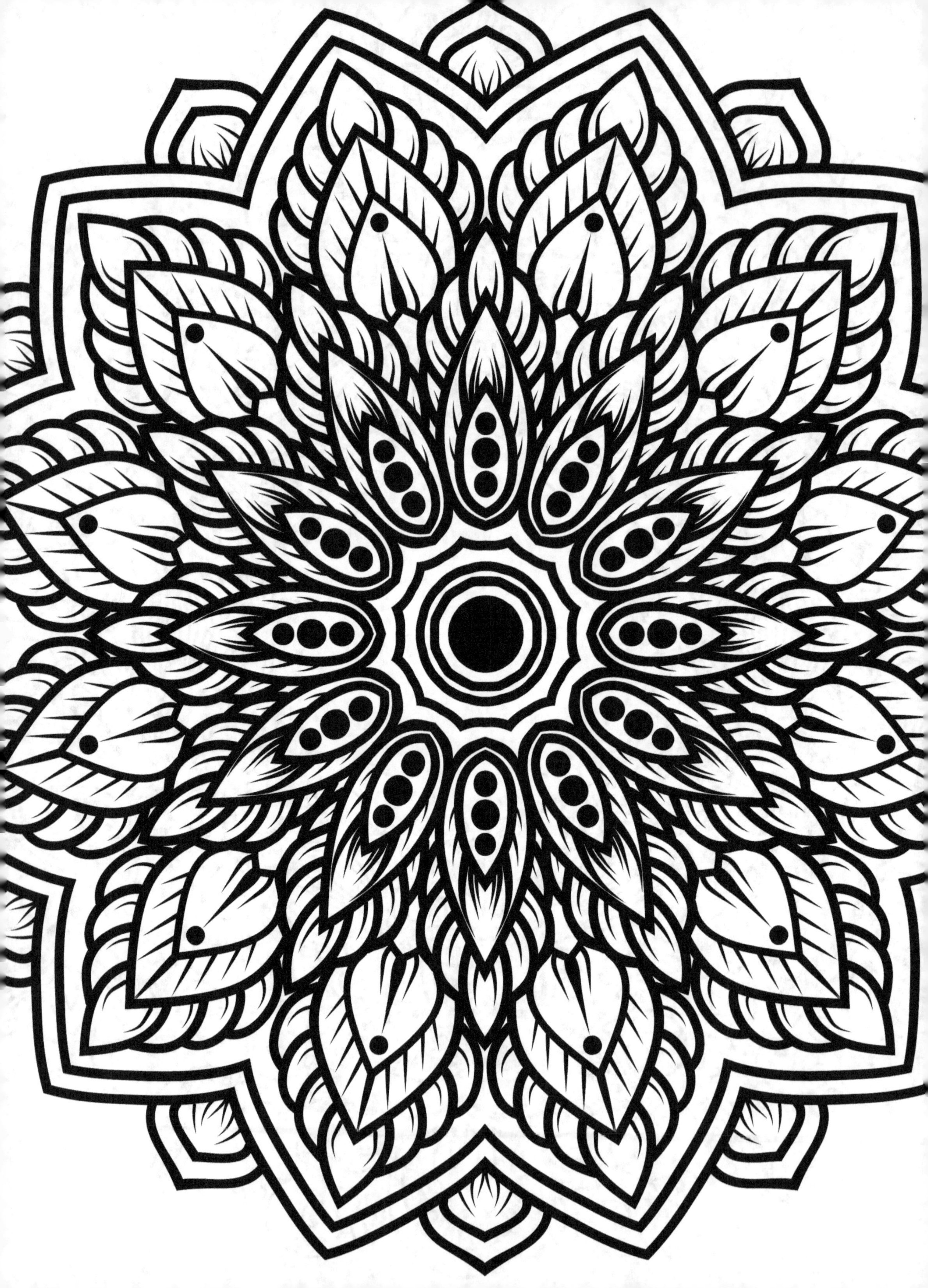

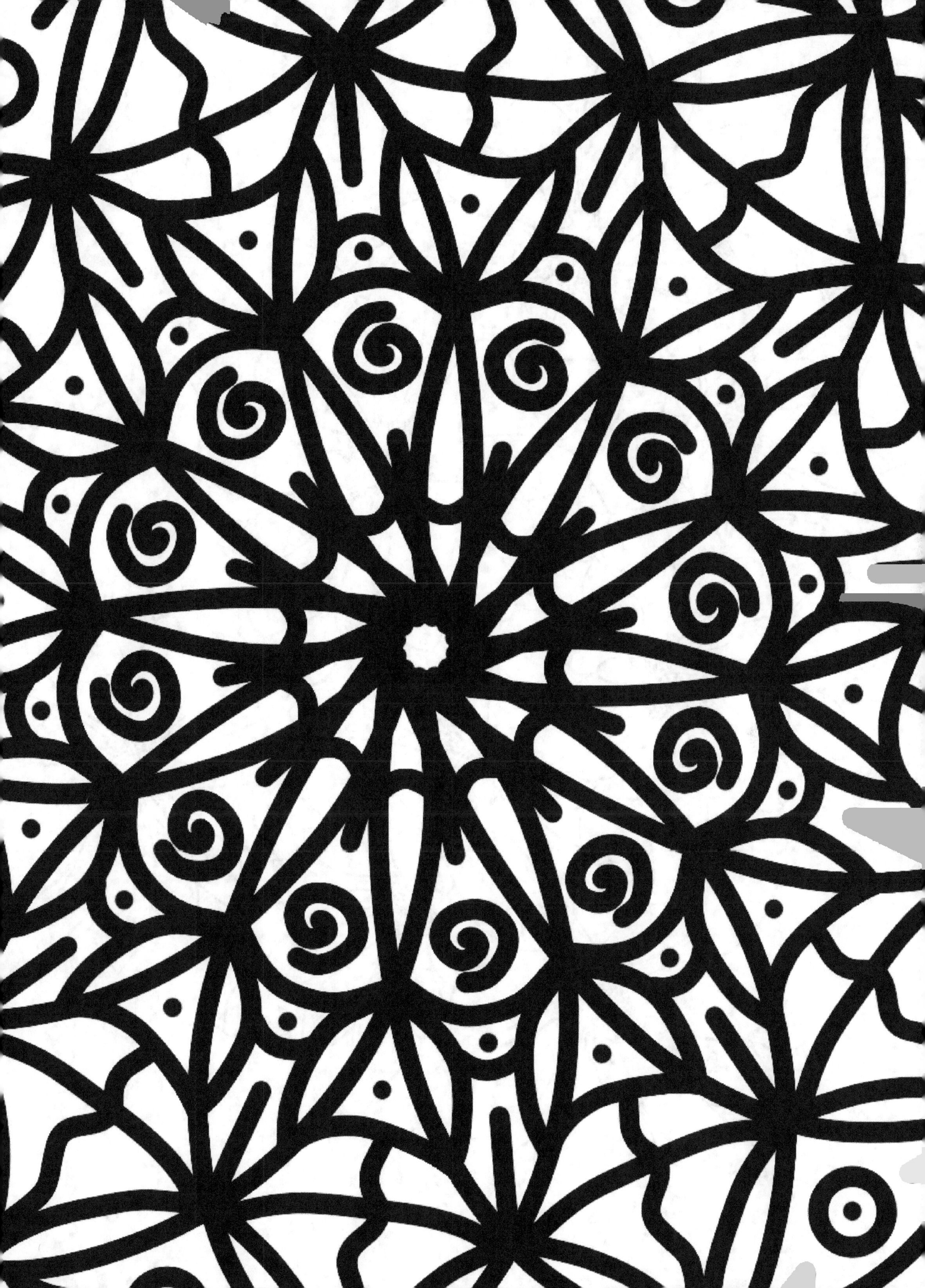

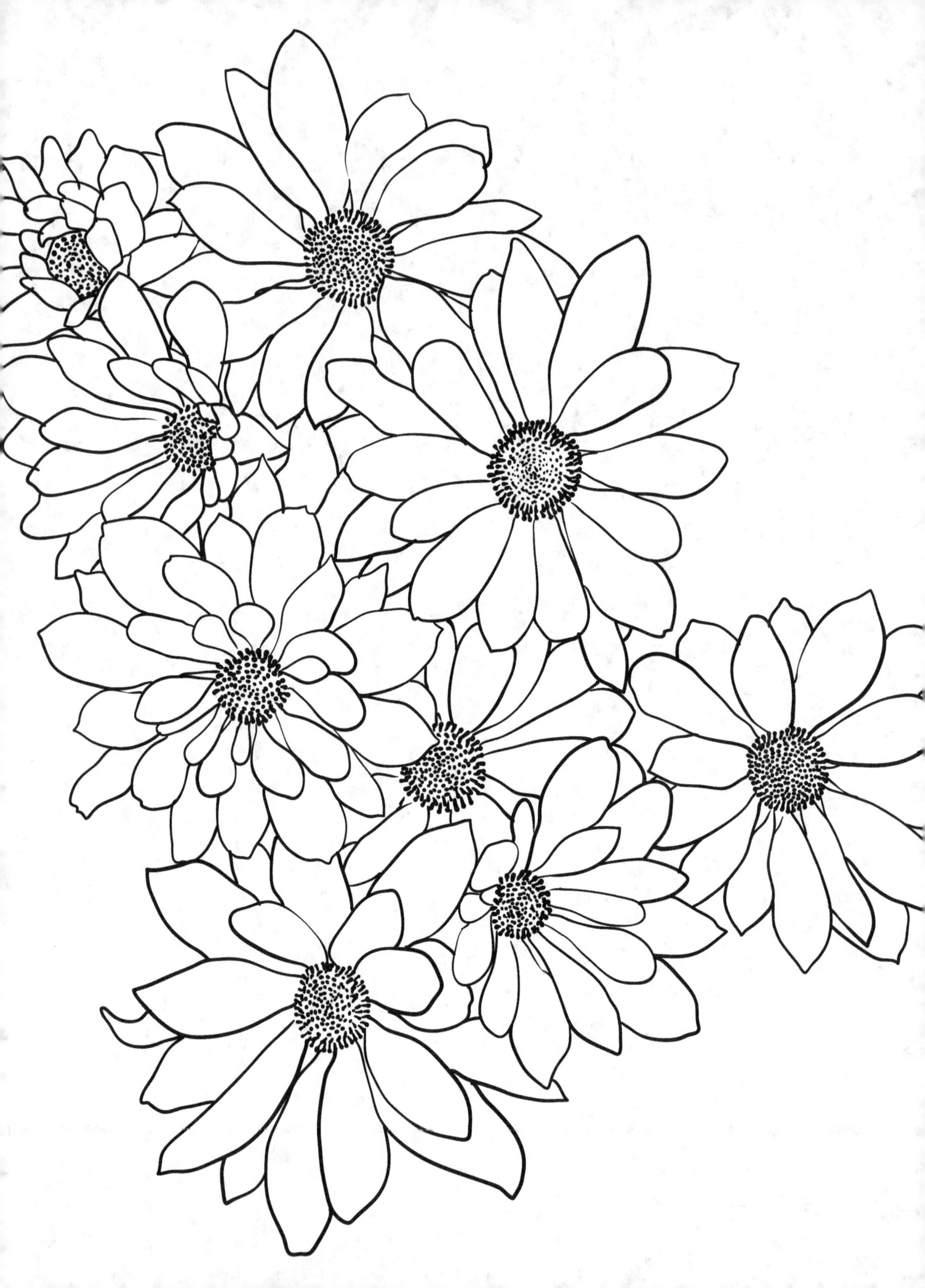

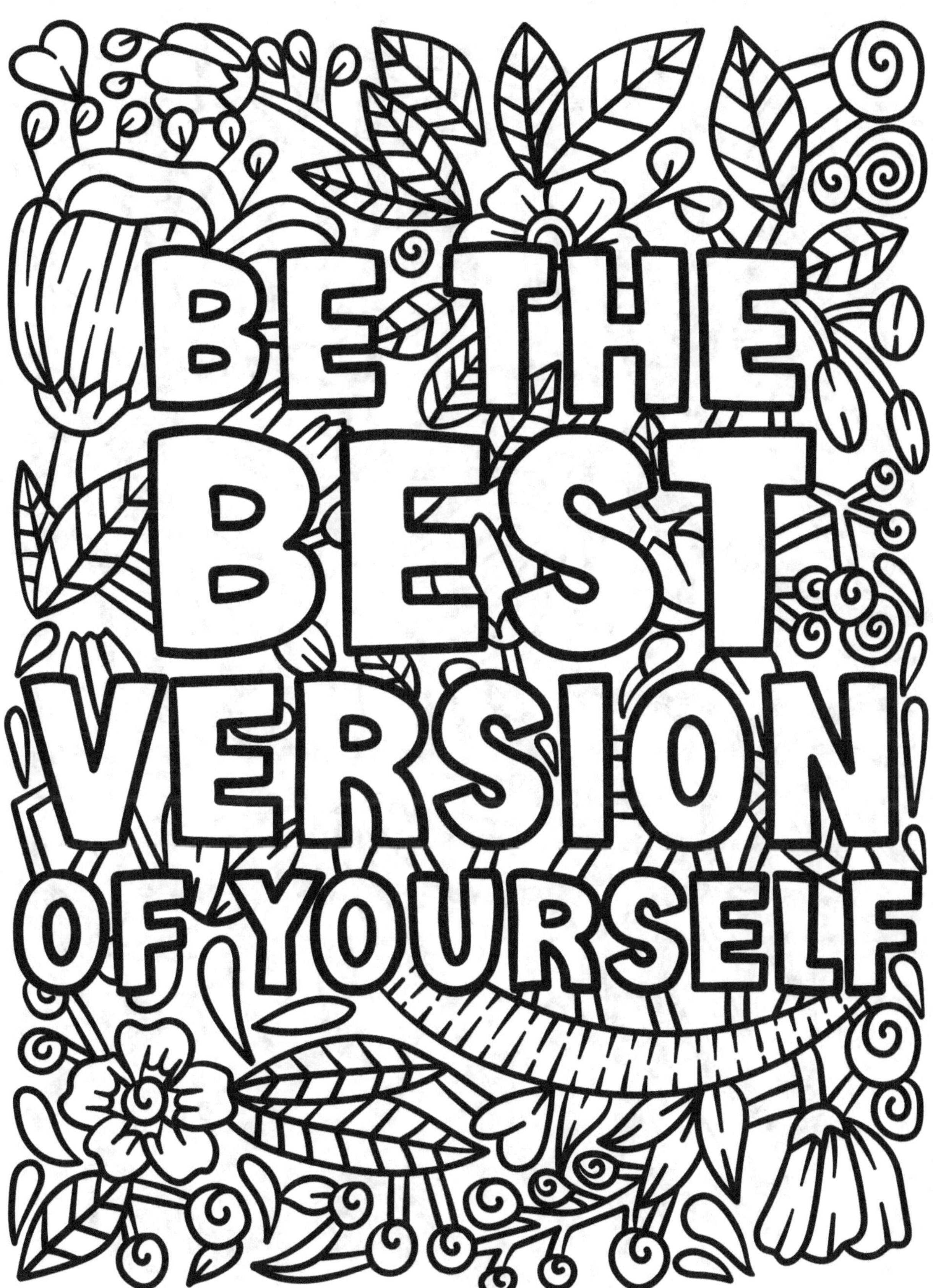

BE THE
BEST
VERSION
OF YOURSELF

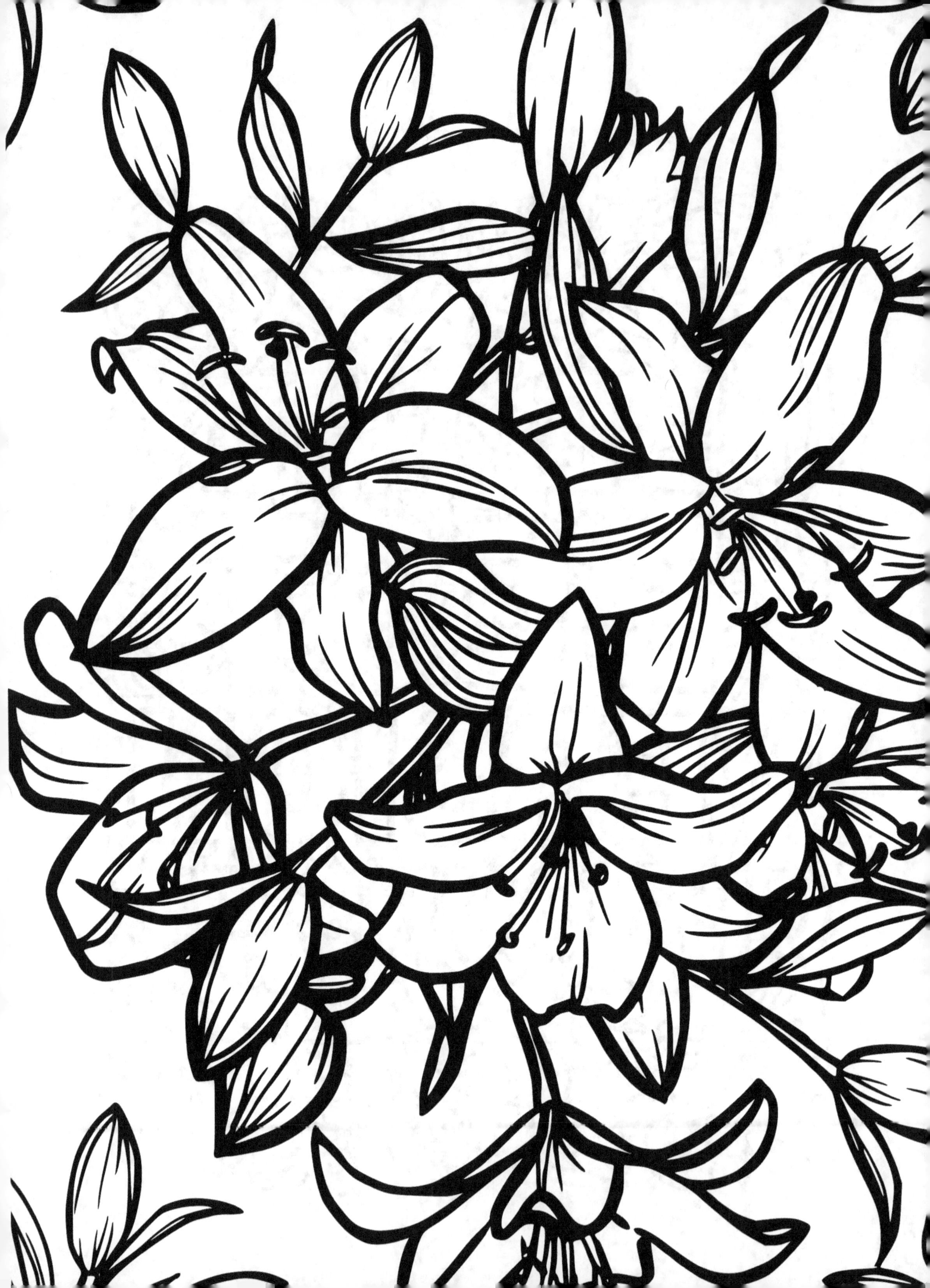

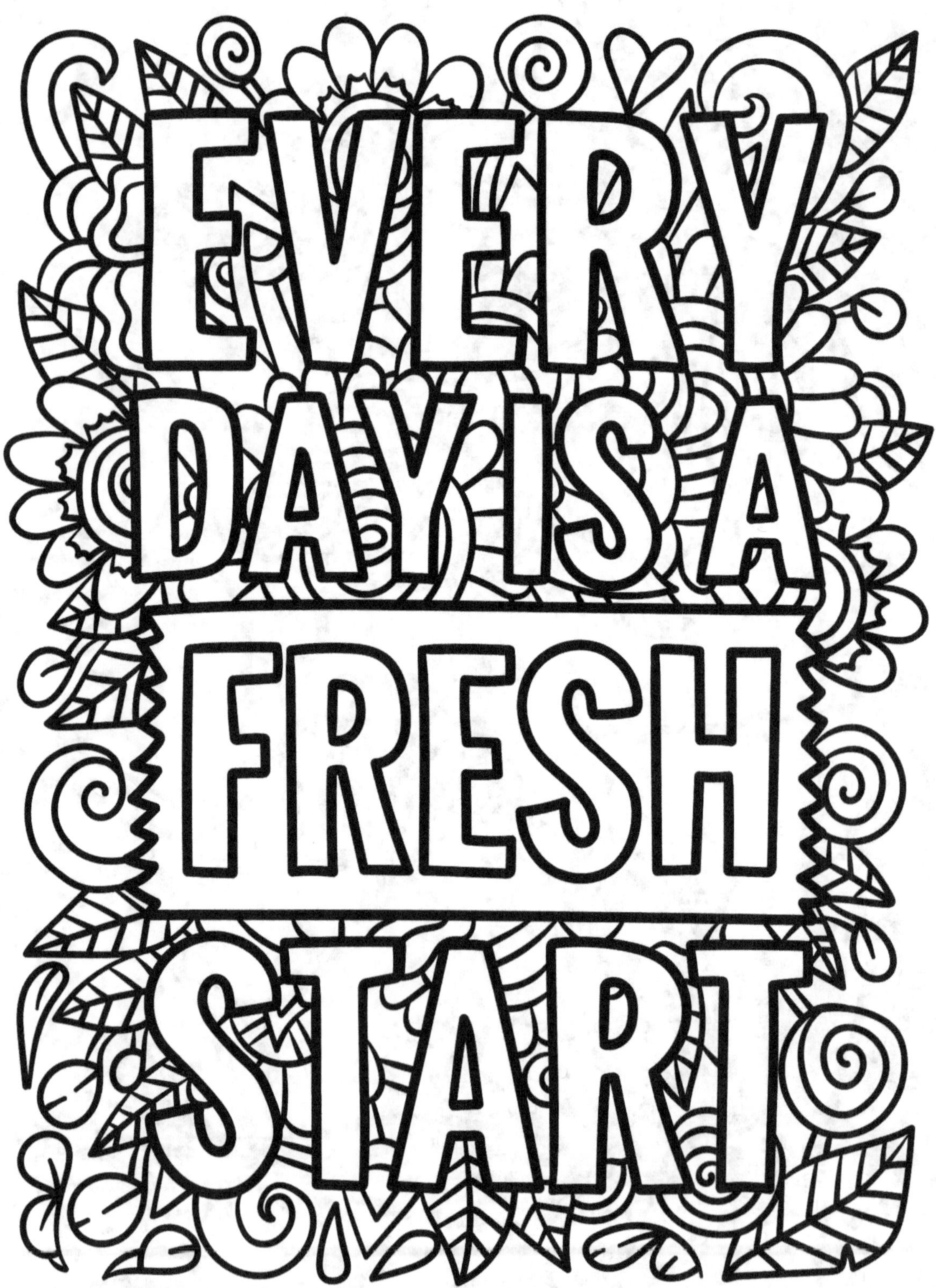

EVERY
DAY IS A
FRESH
START

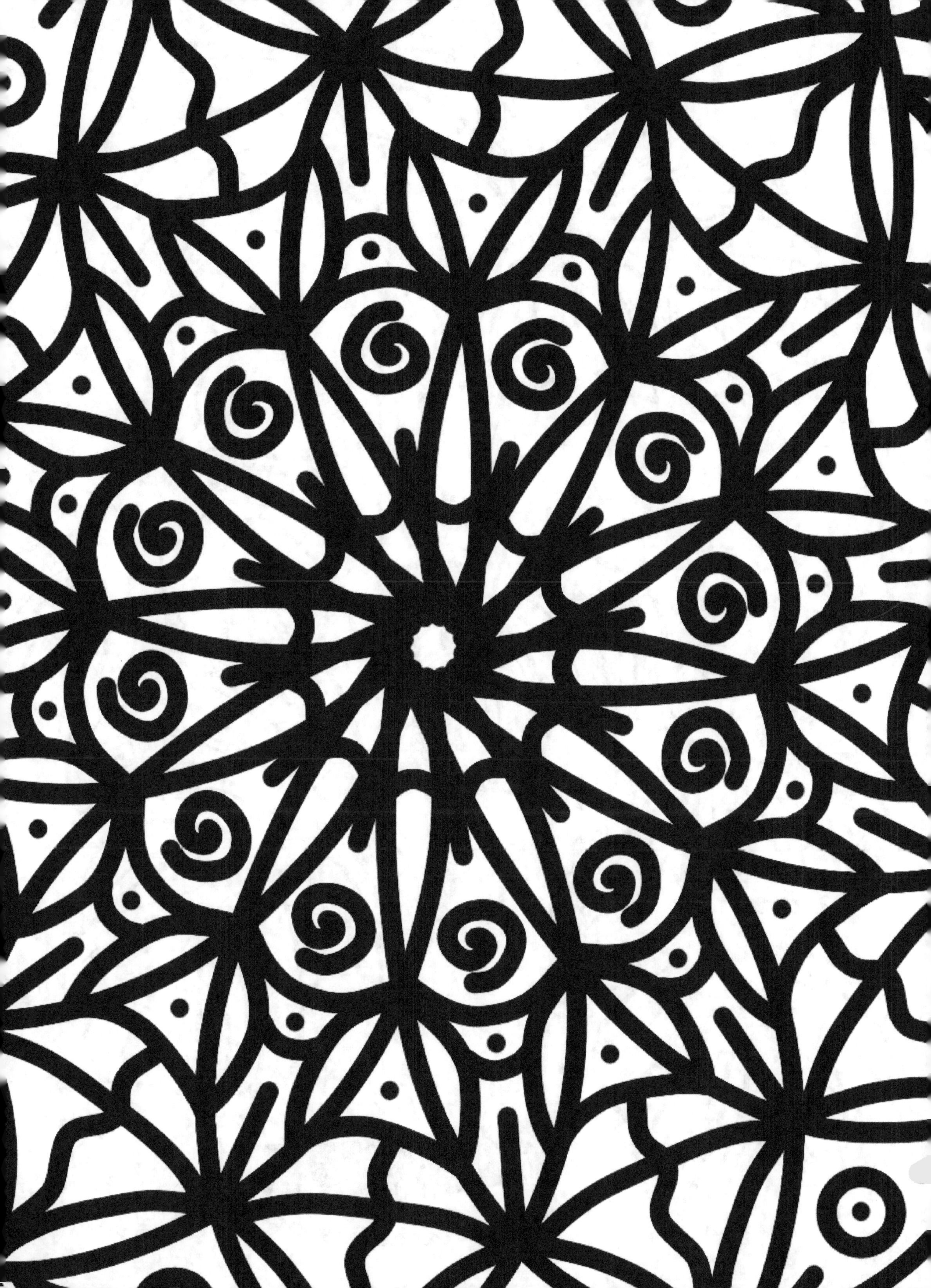

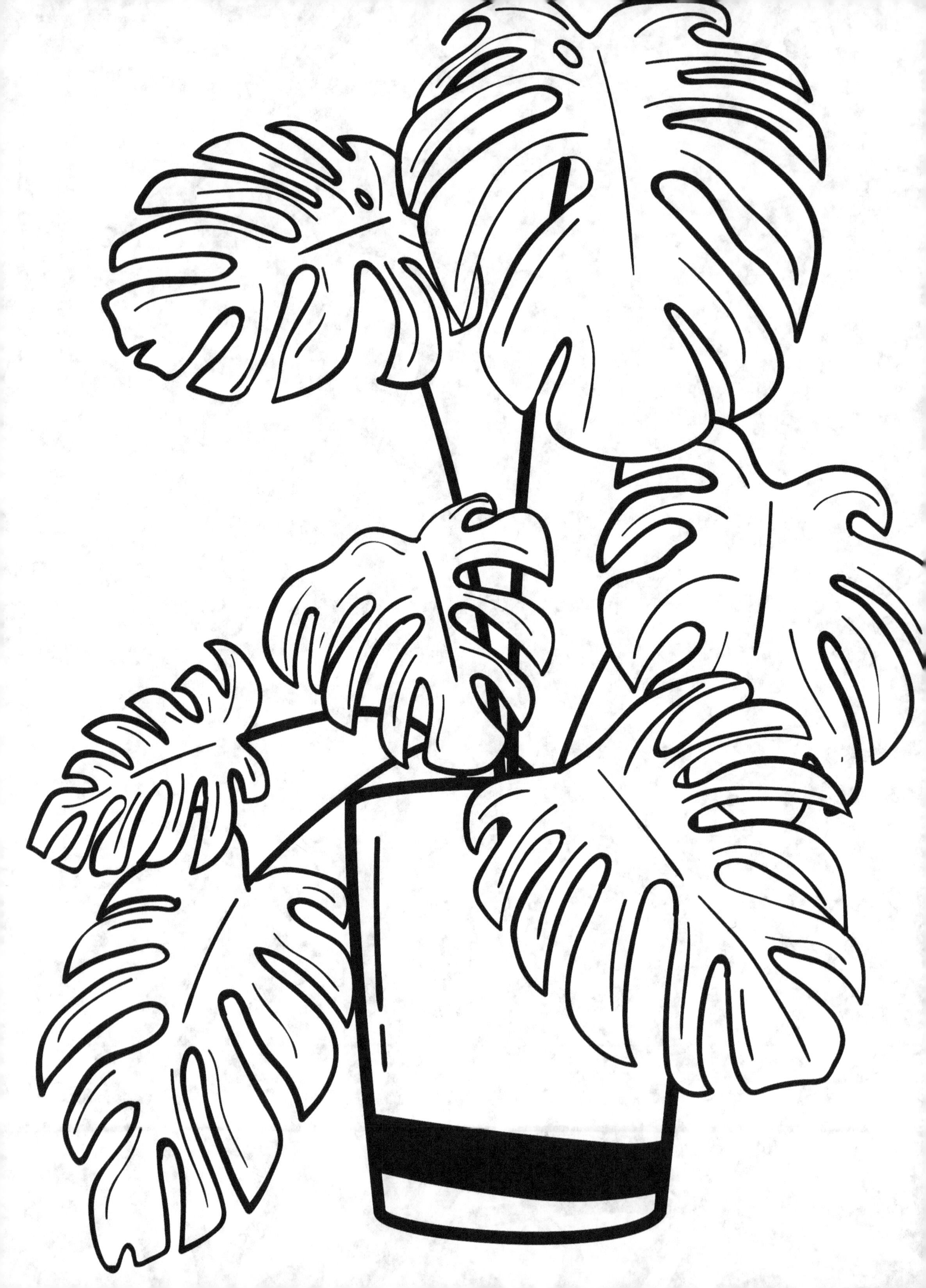

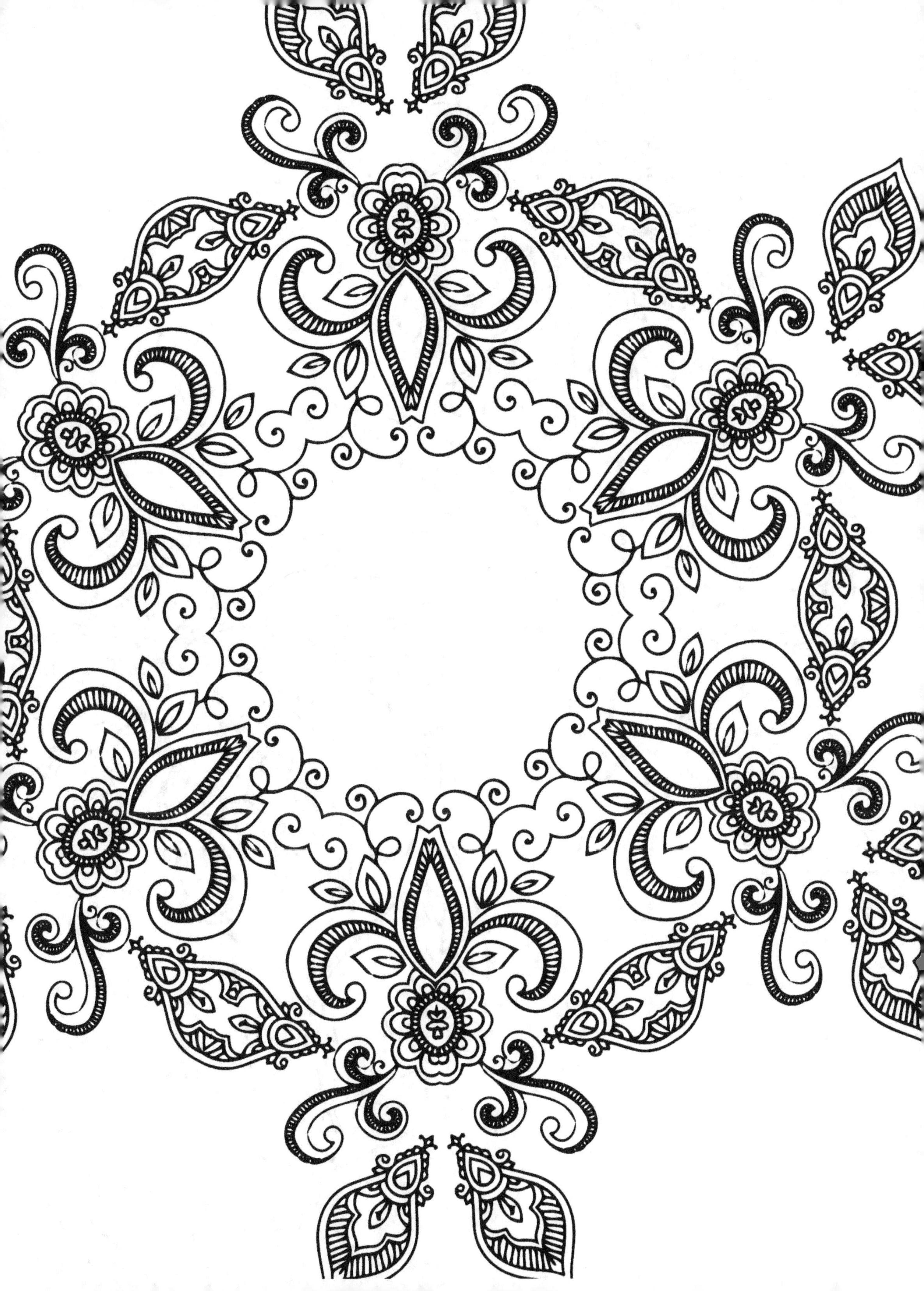

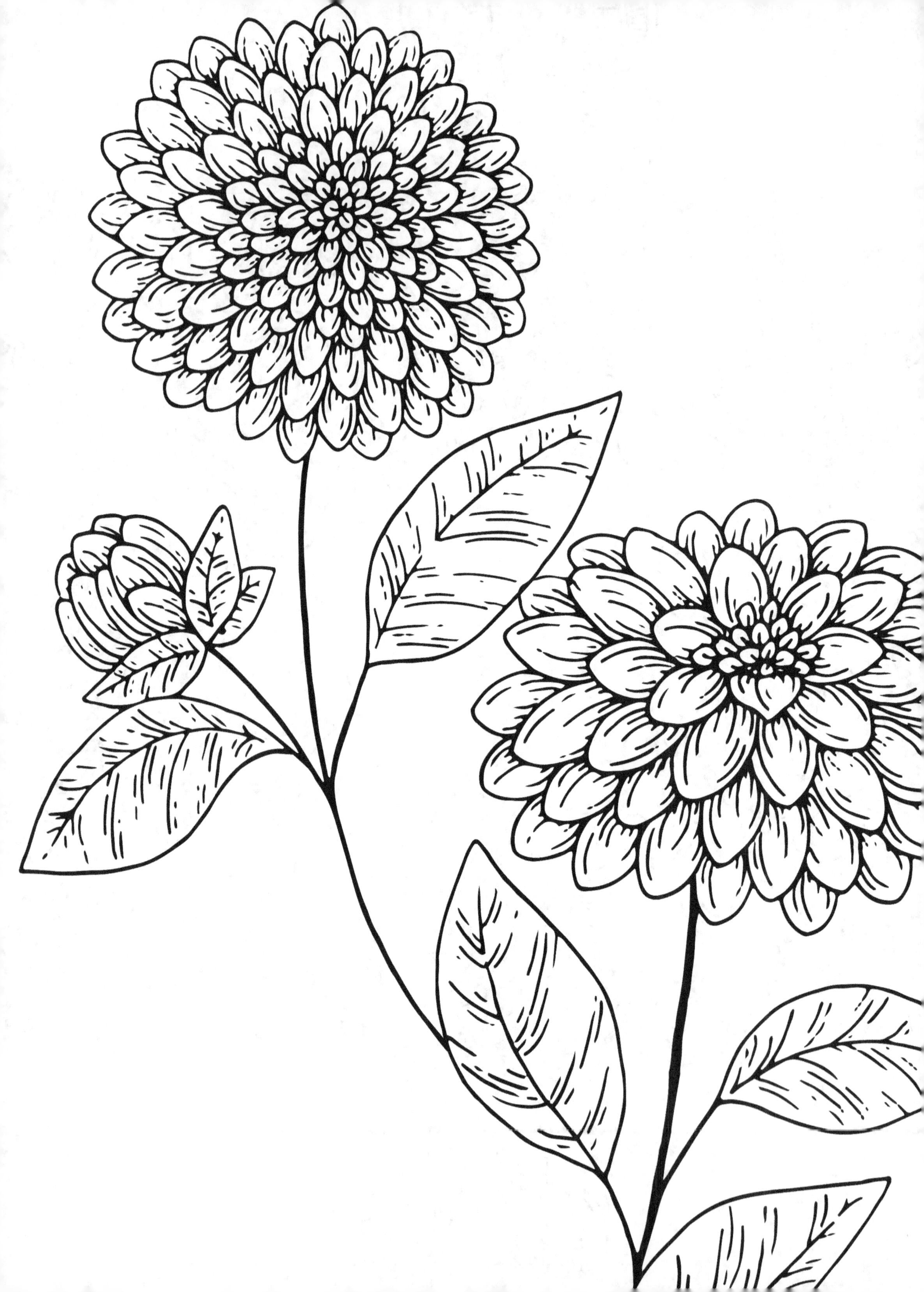

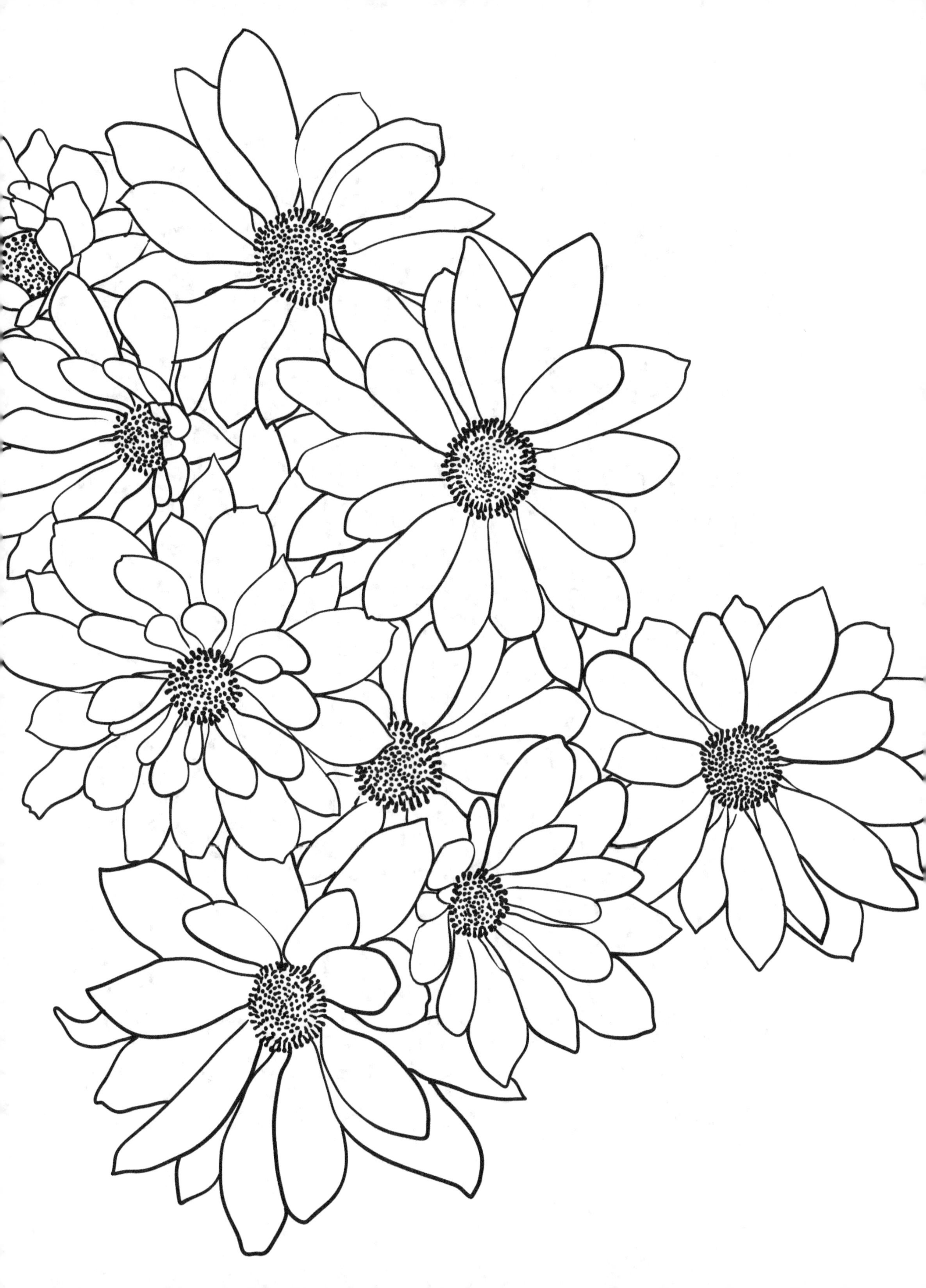

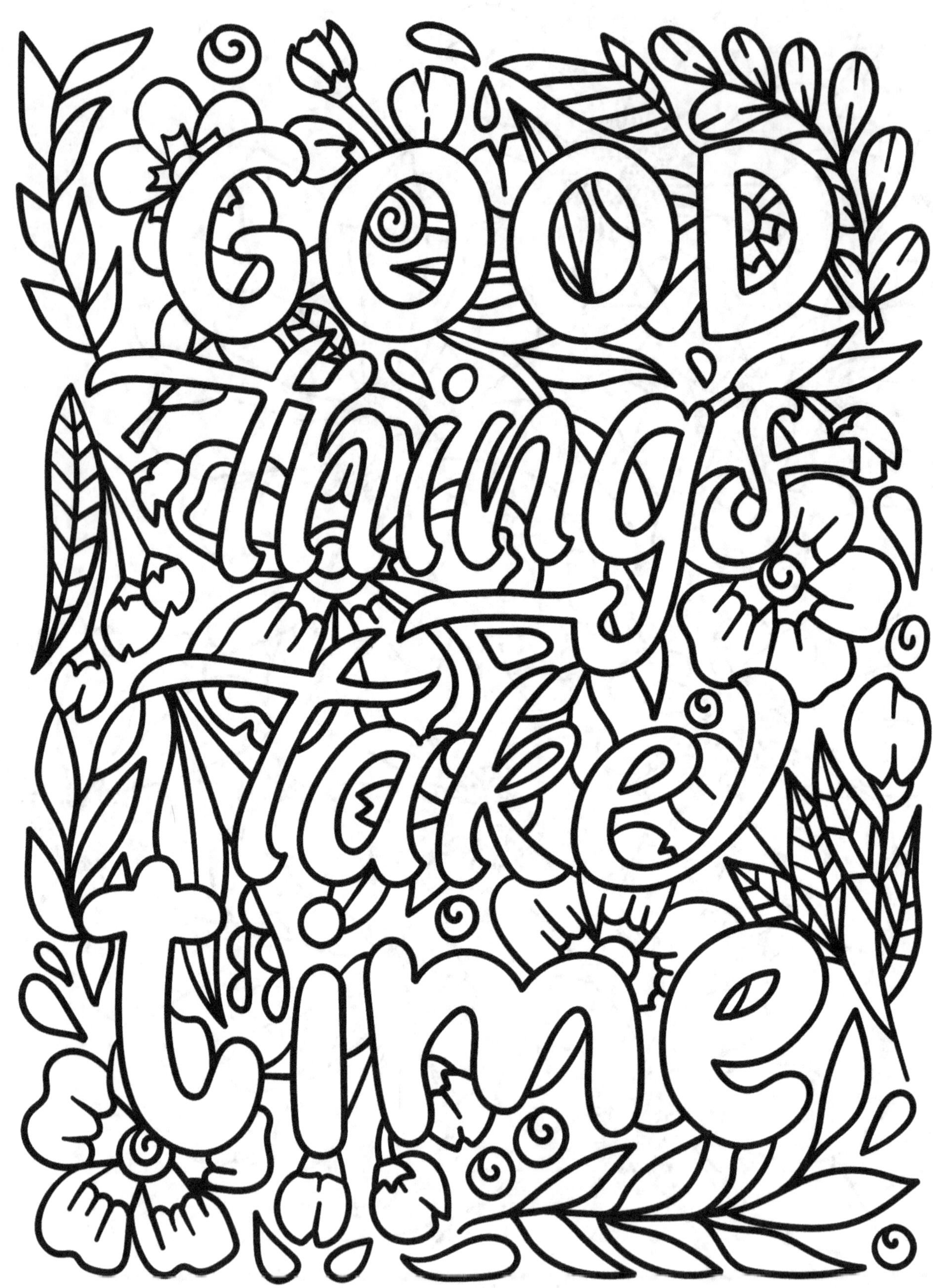

GOOD
things
take
time

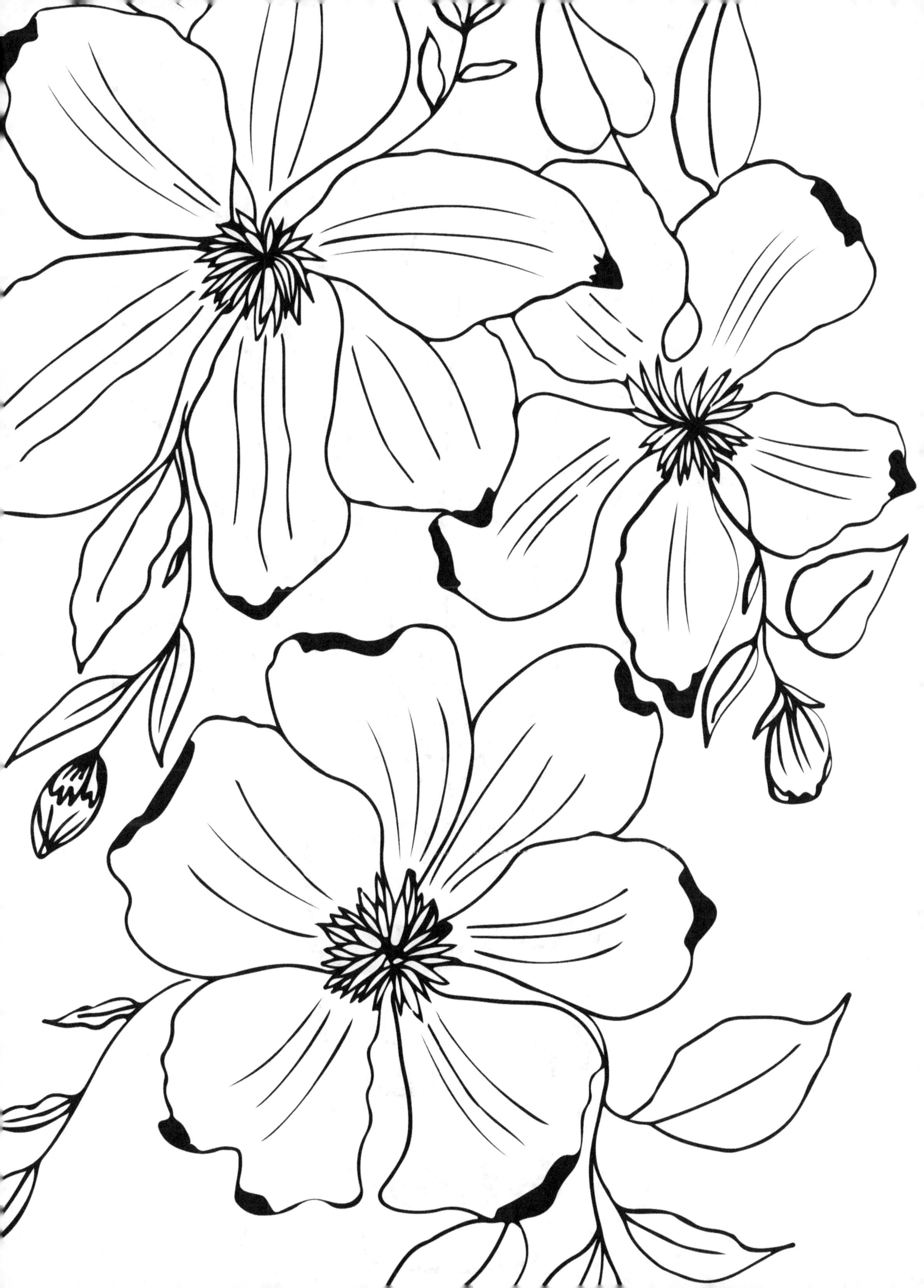

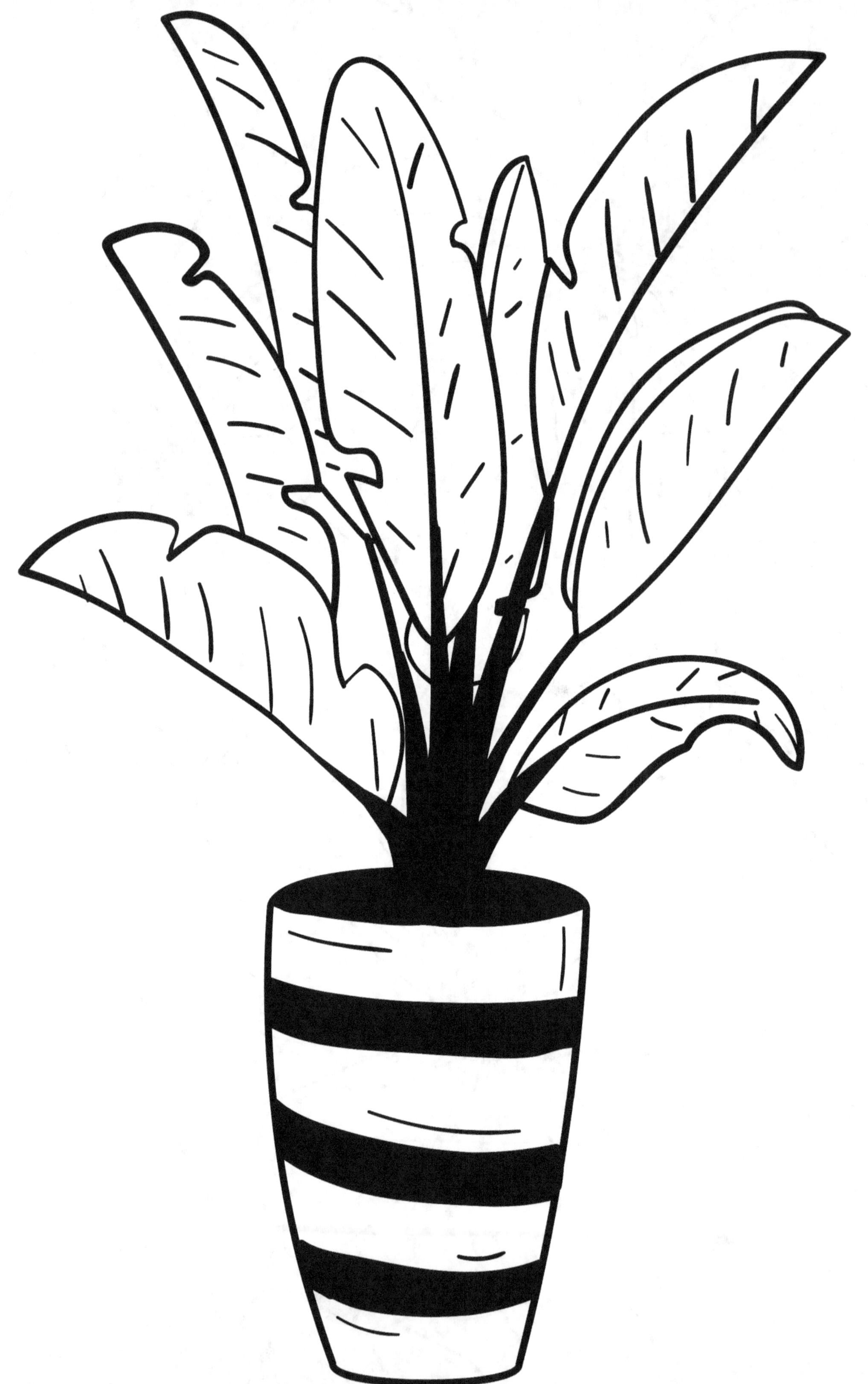

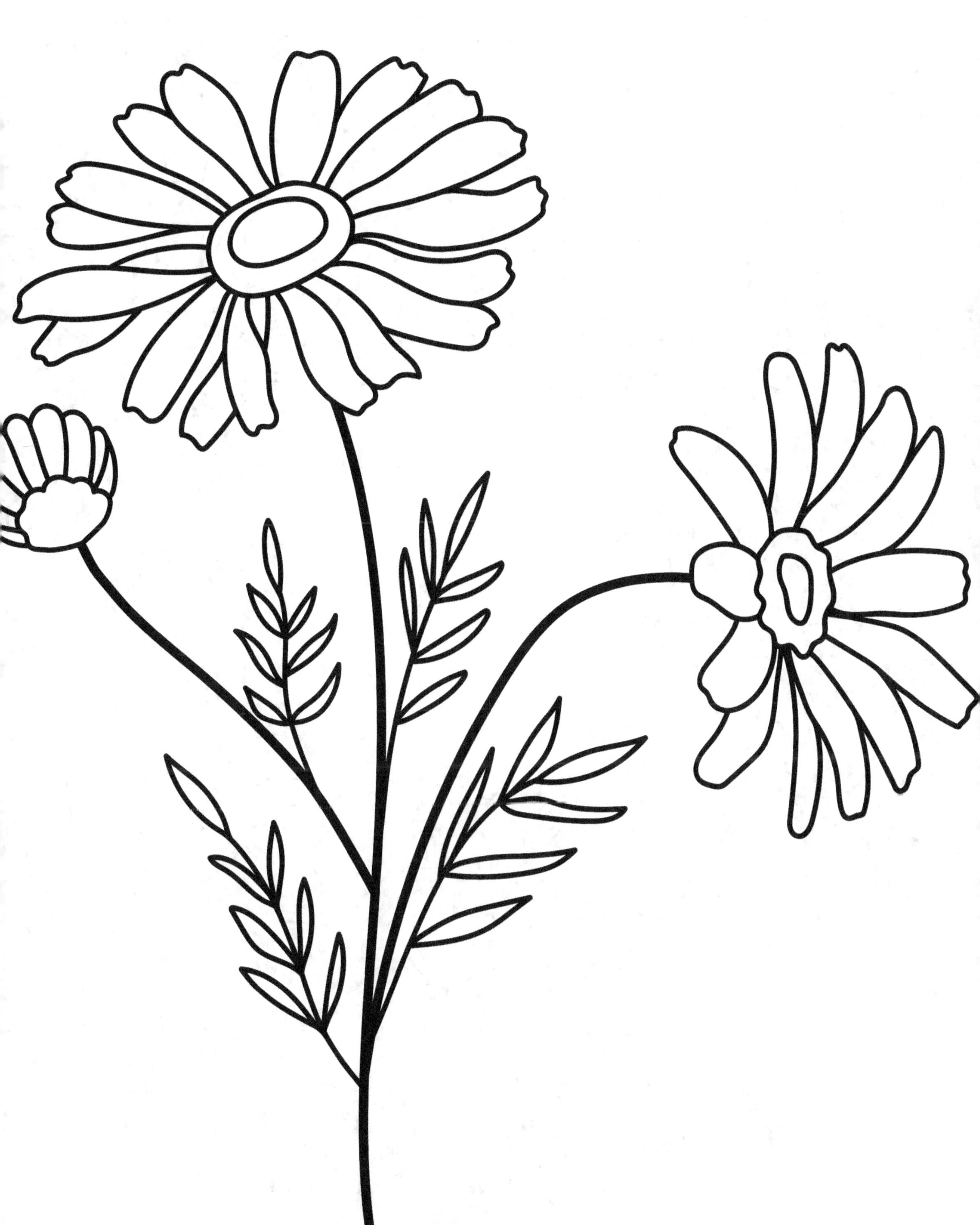

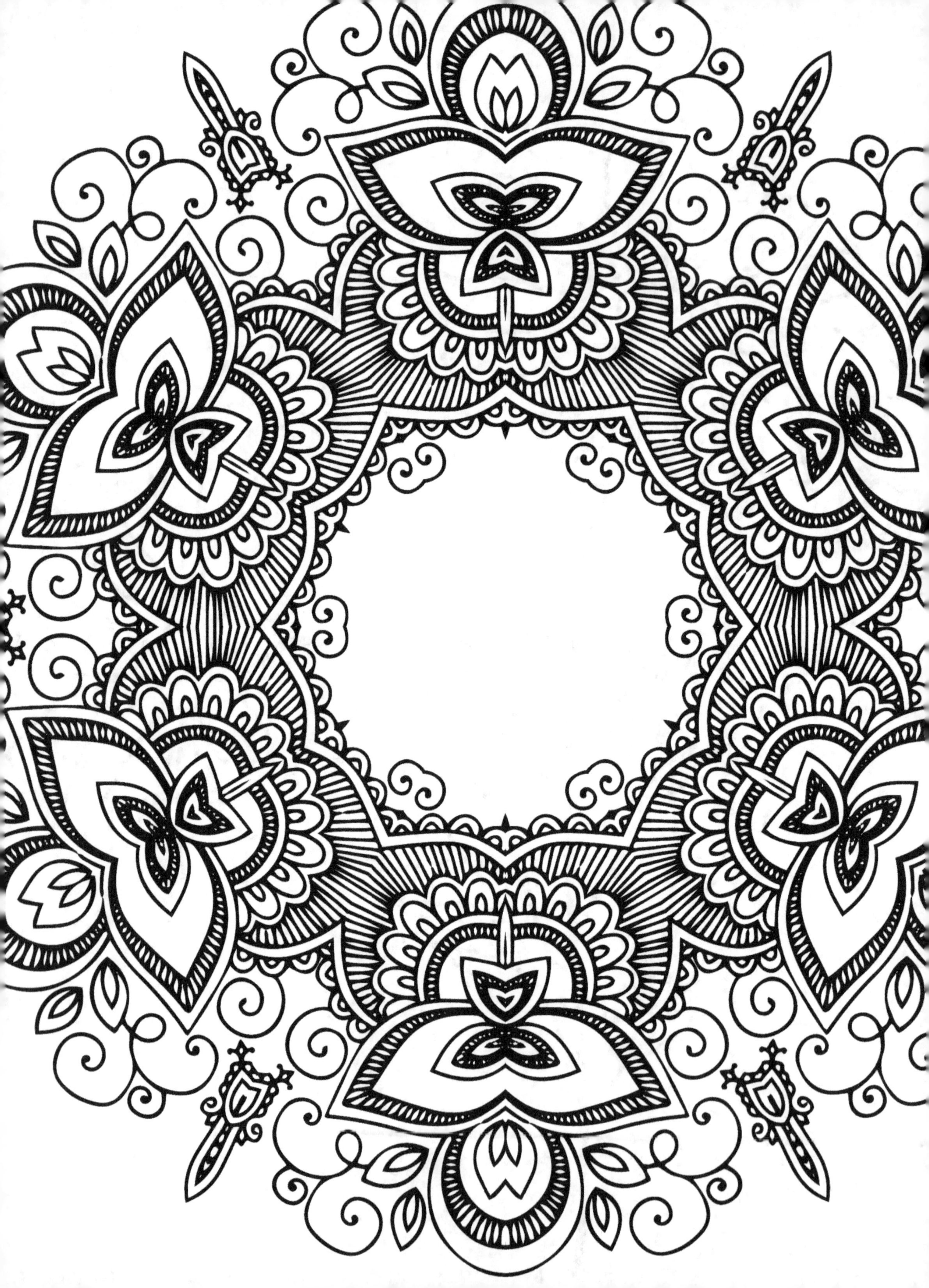

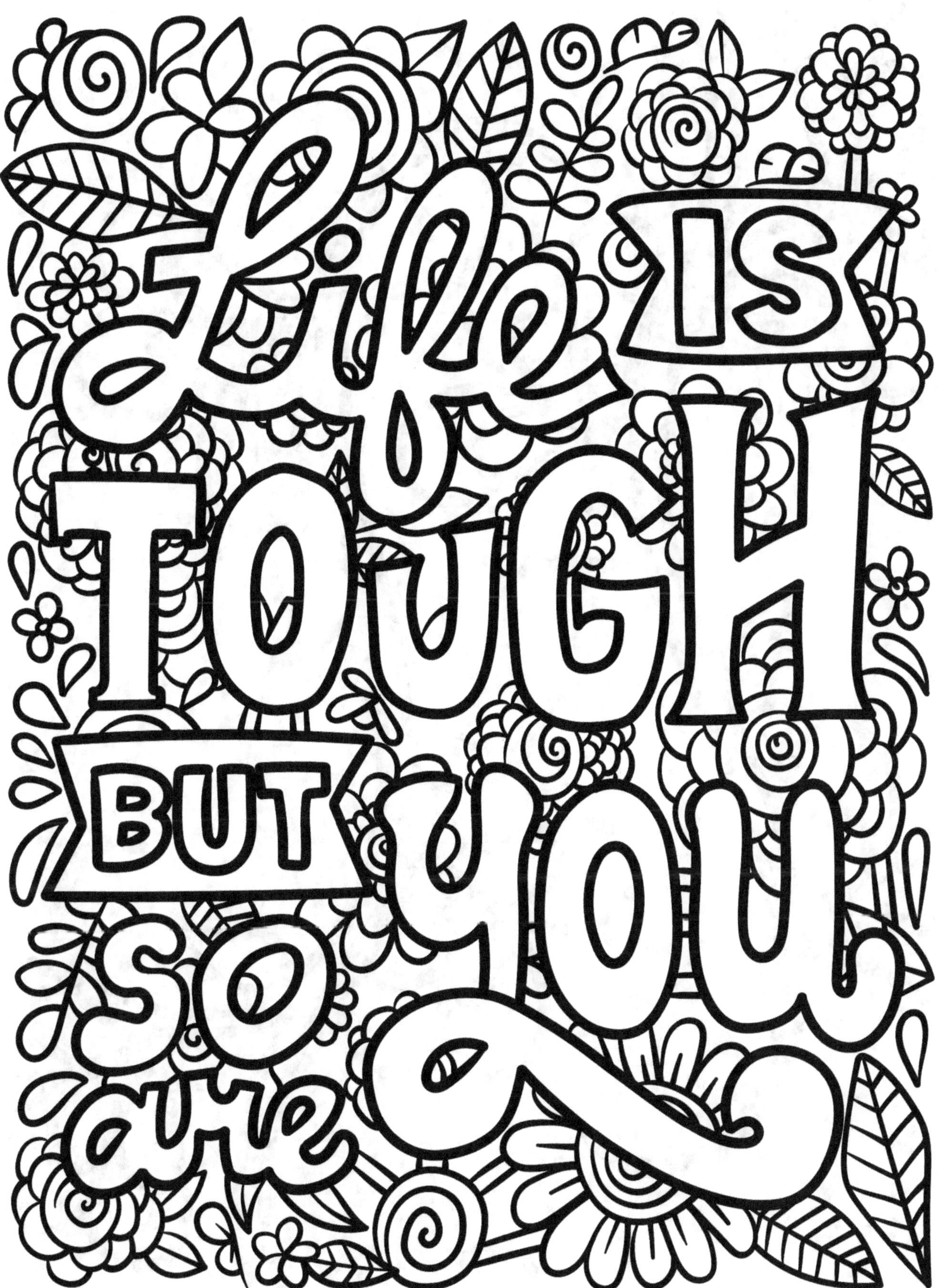
Life is
Tough
but
so
are
you

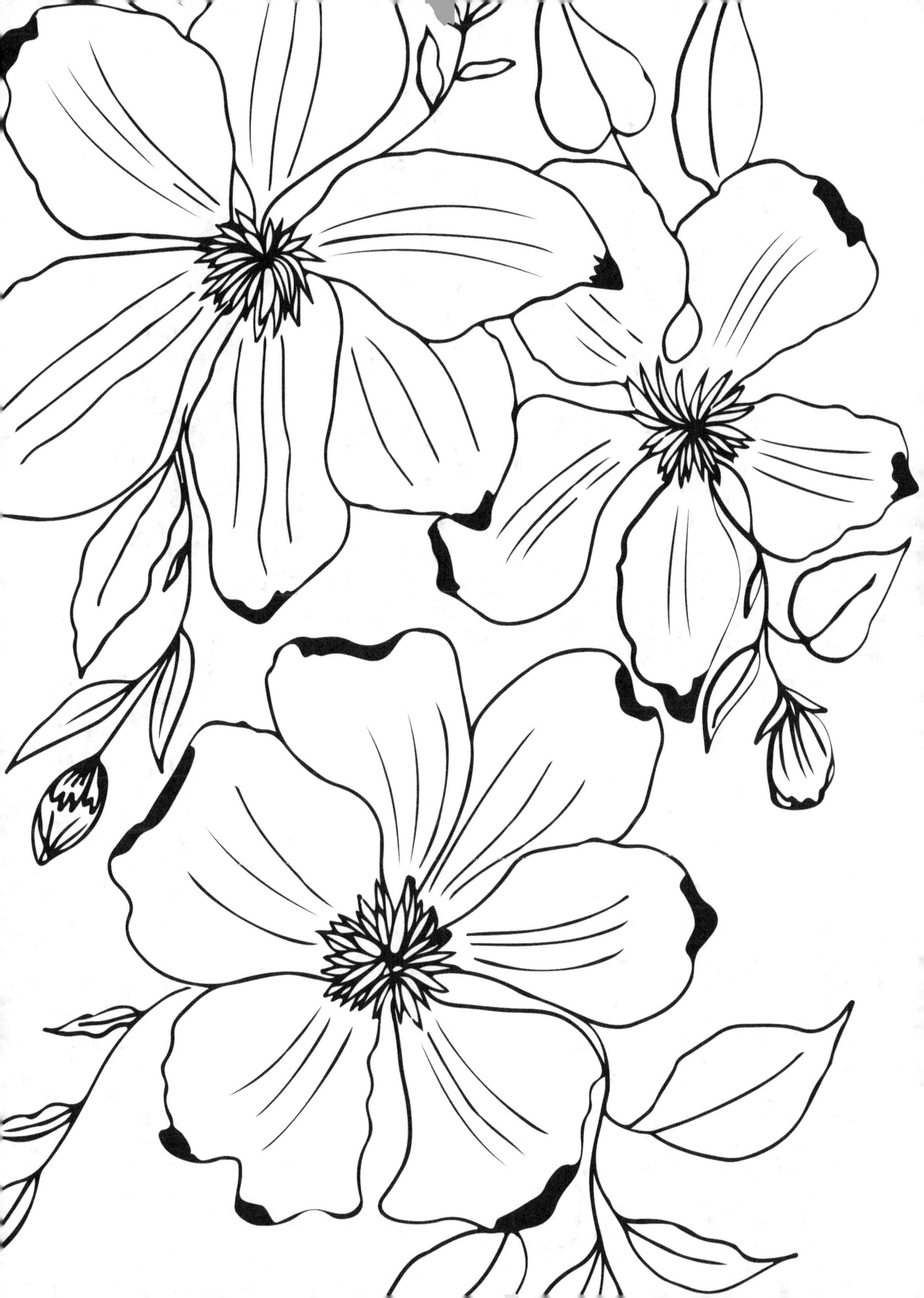

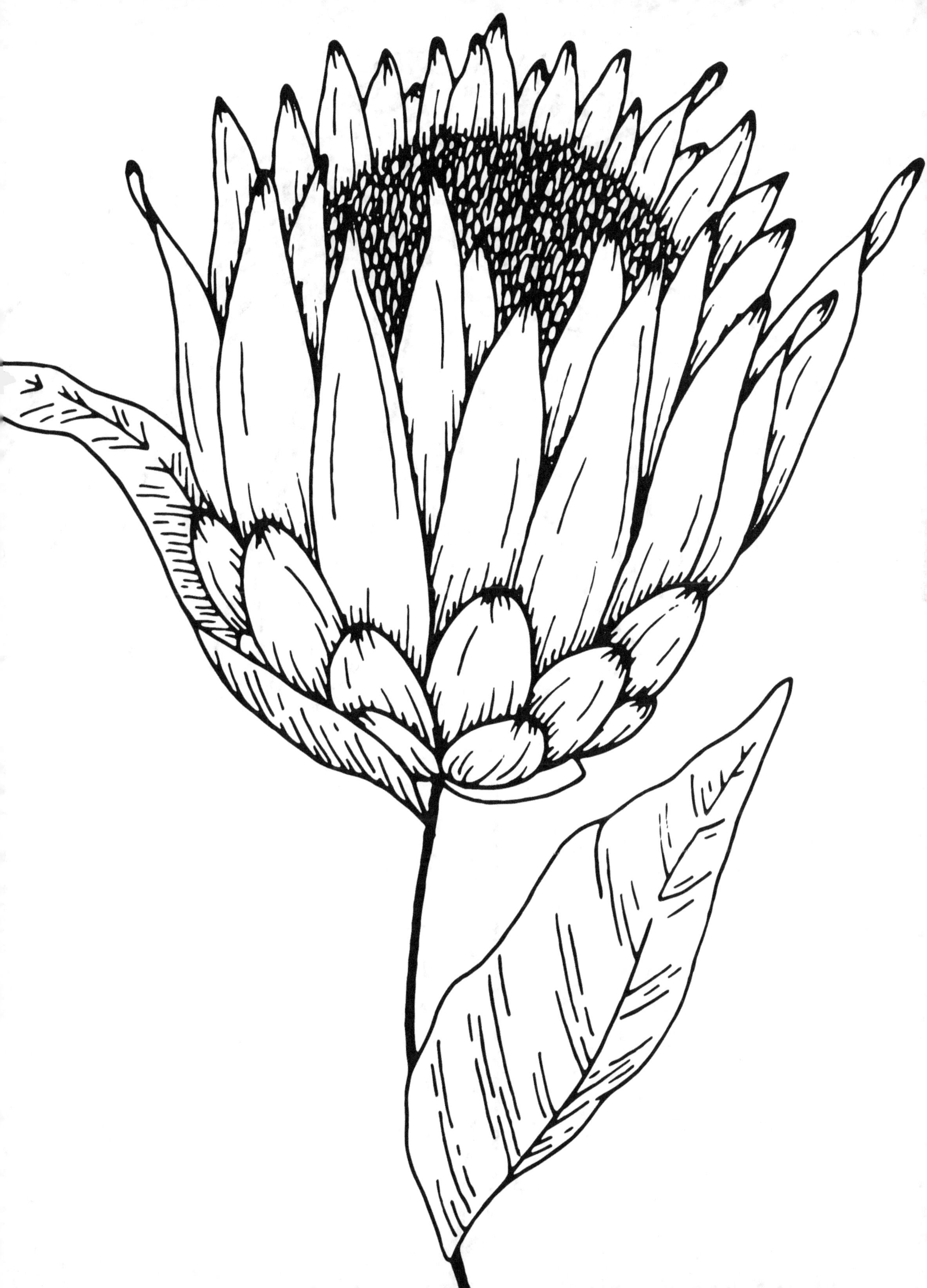

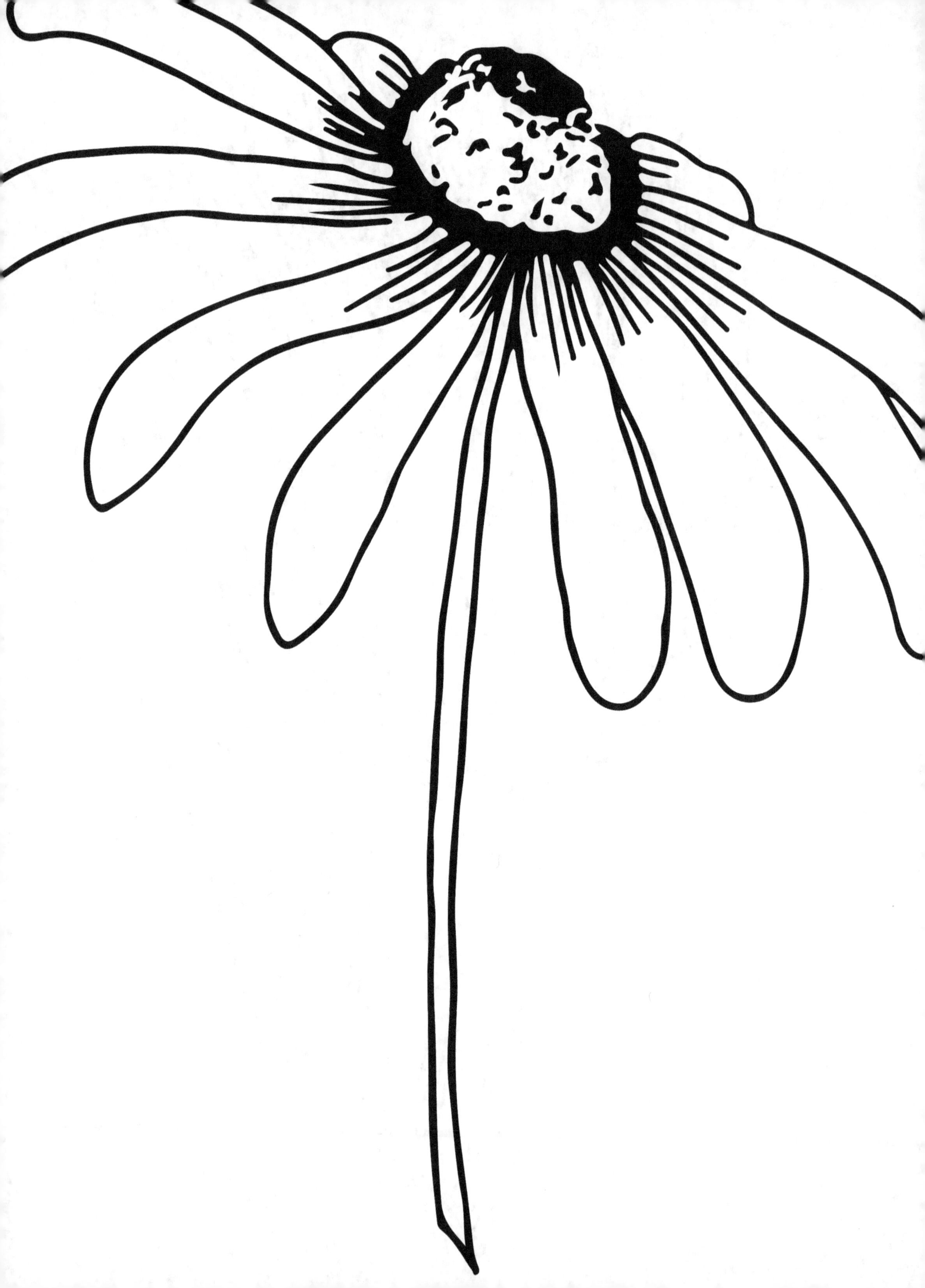

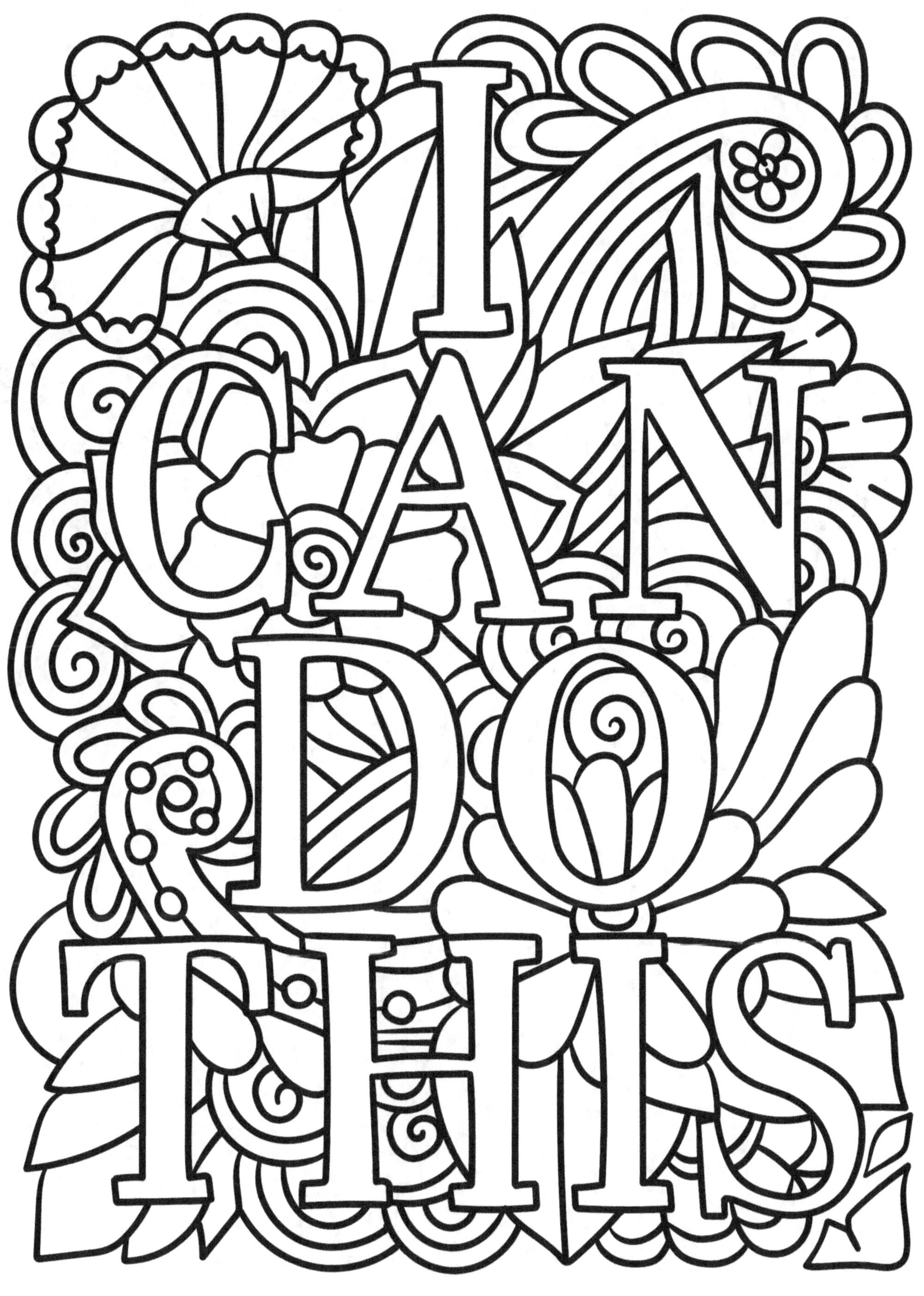
I CAN DO THIS

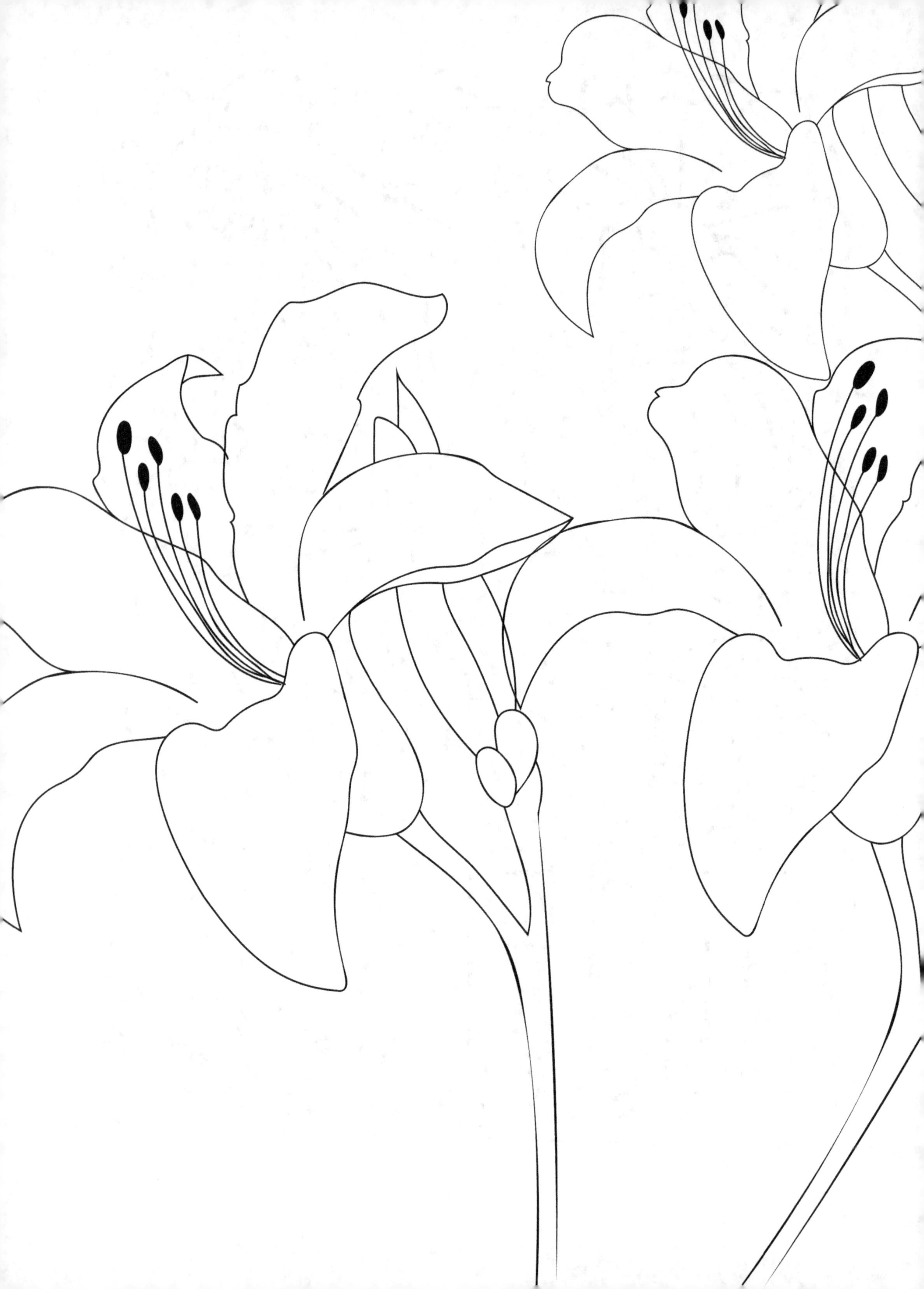

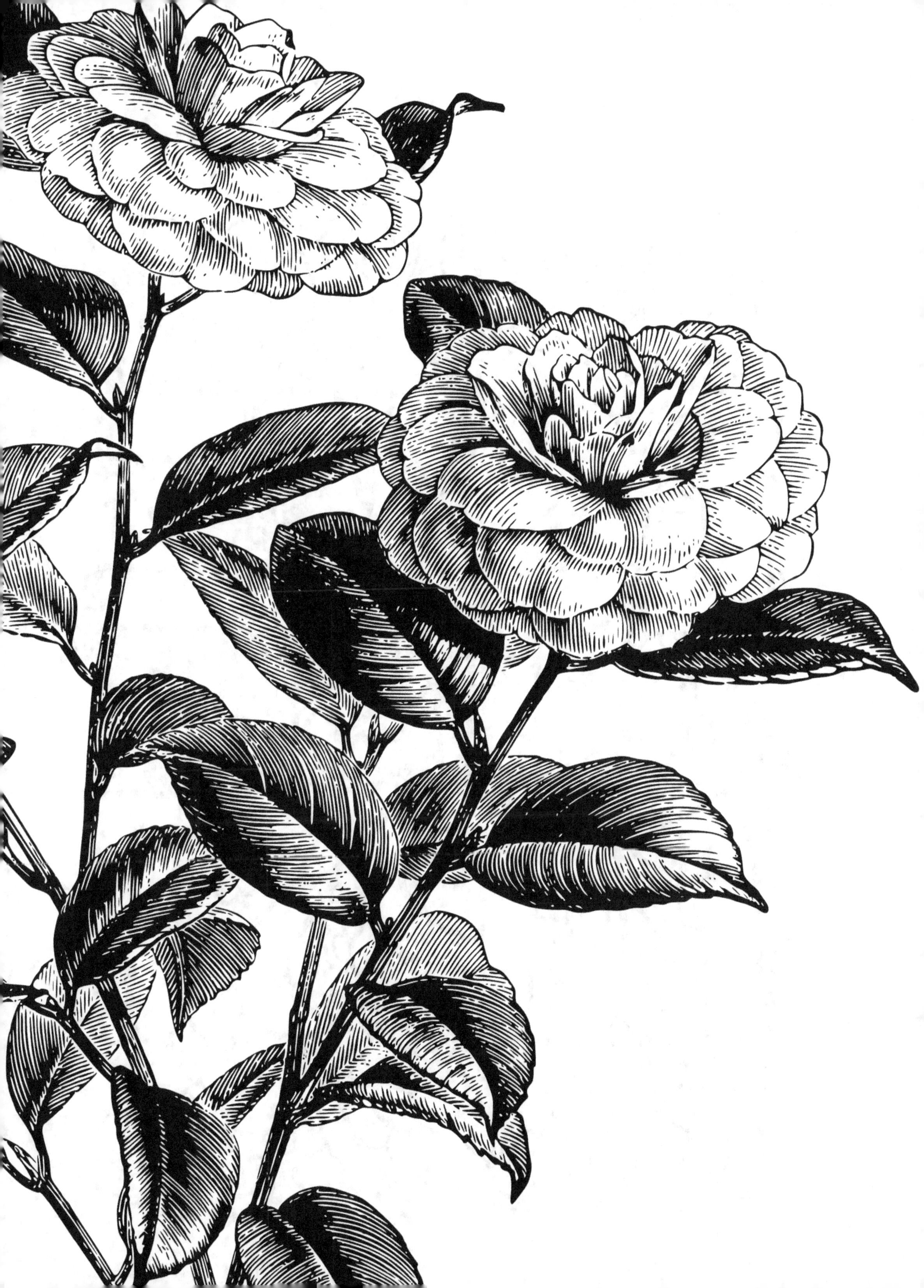

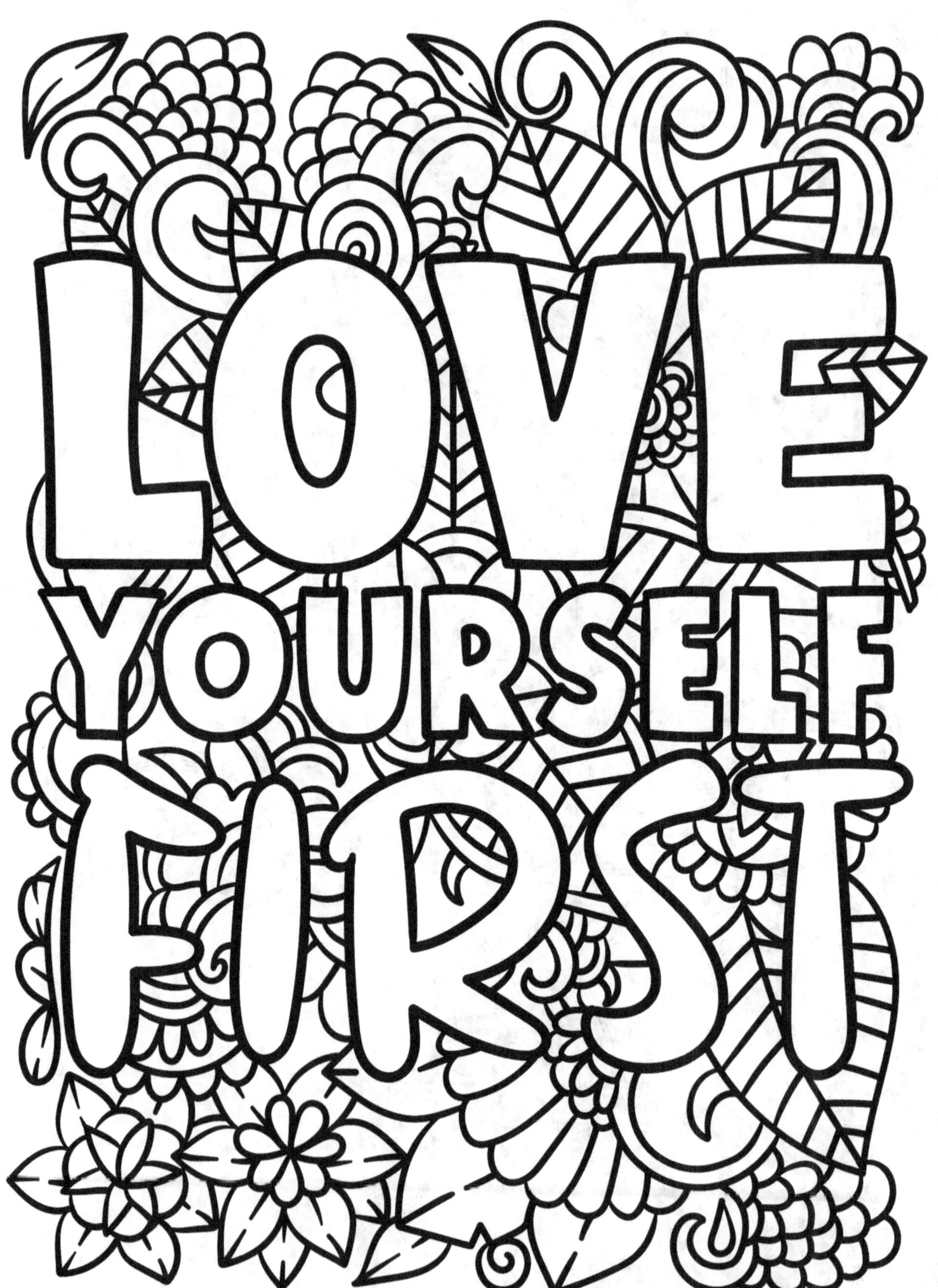

LOVE
YOURSELF
FIRST

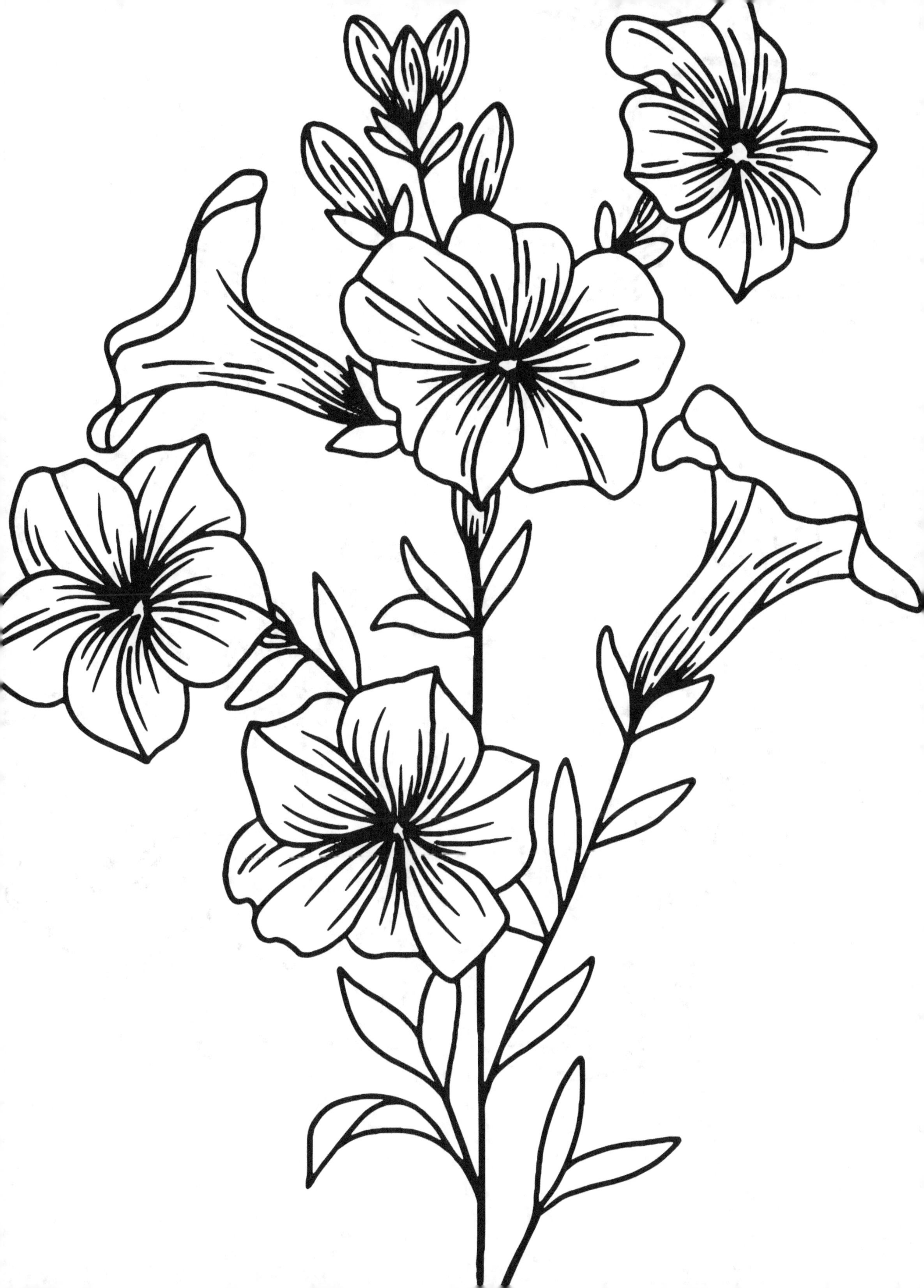

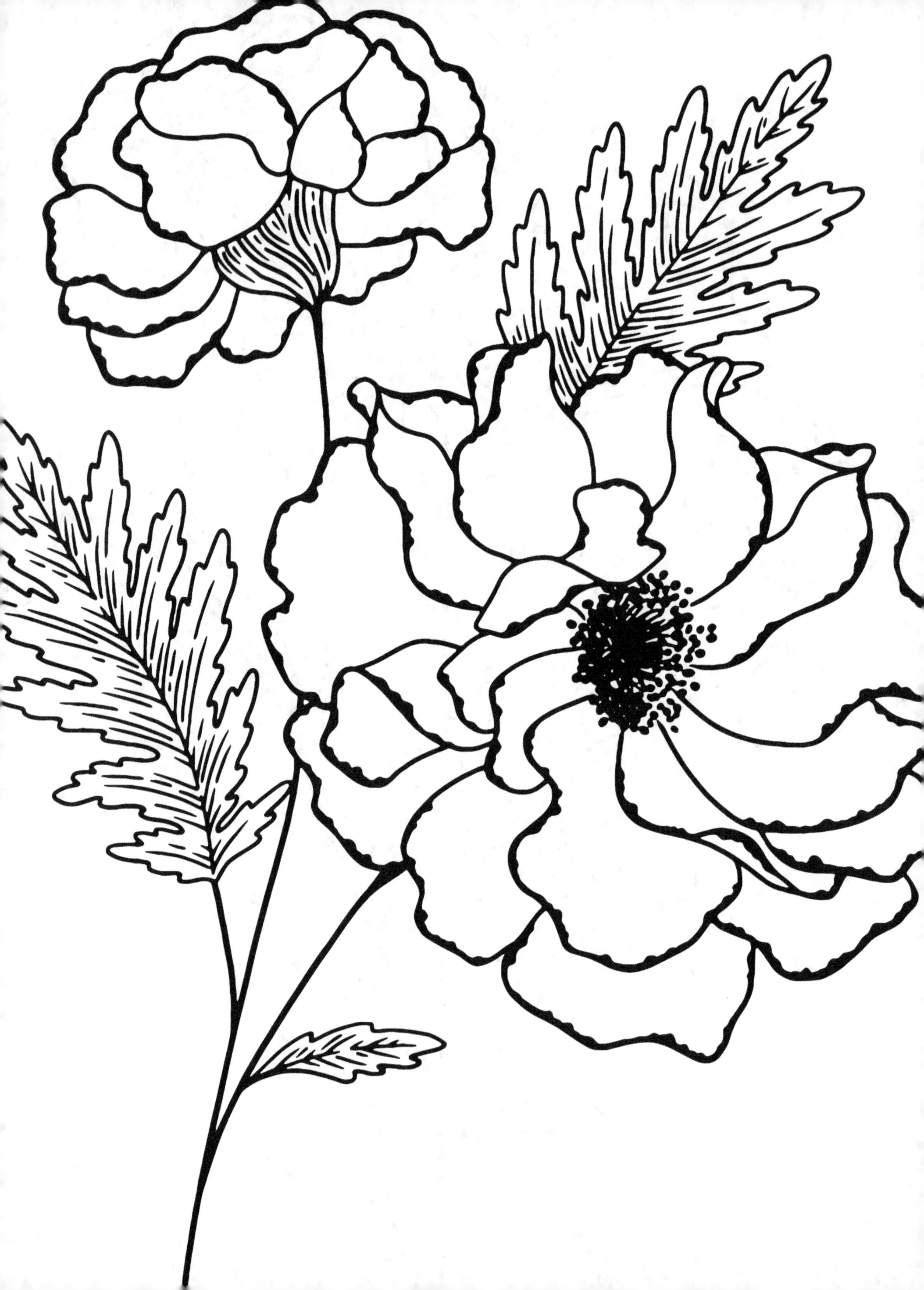

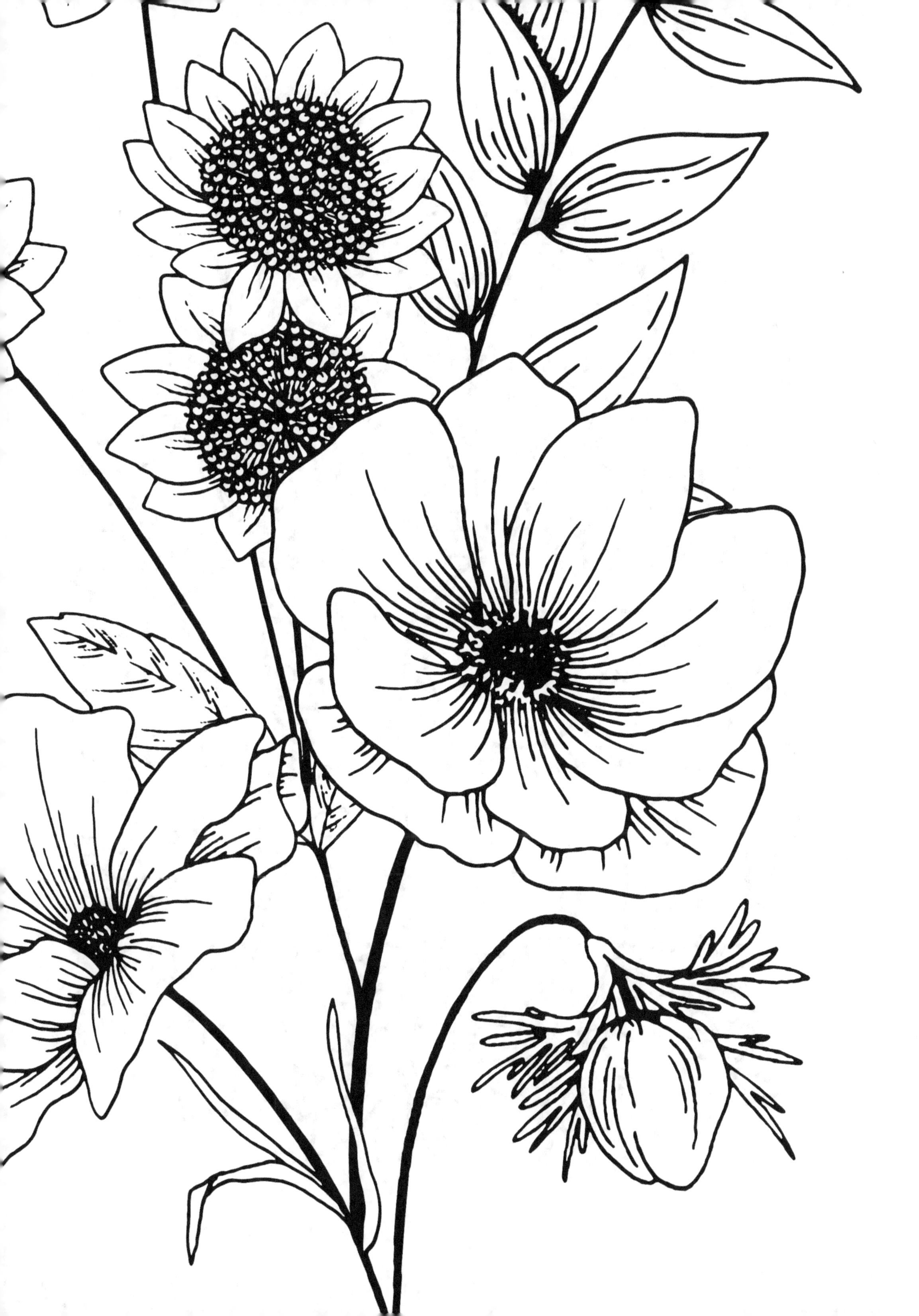

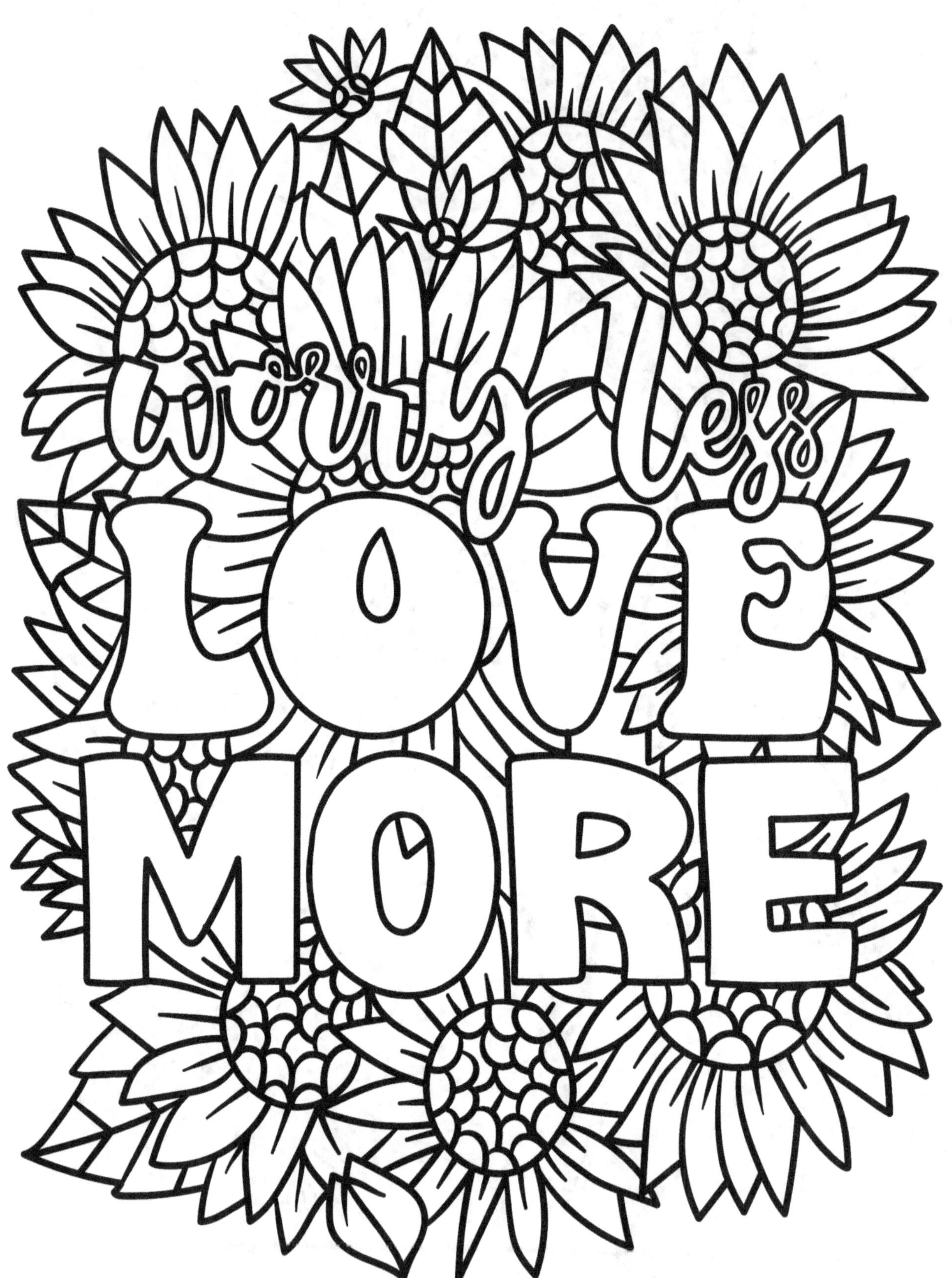

worry less
LOVE
MORE

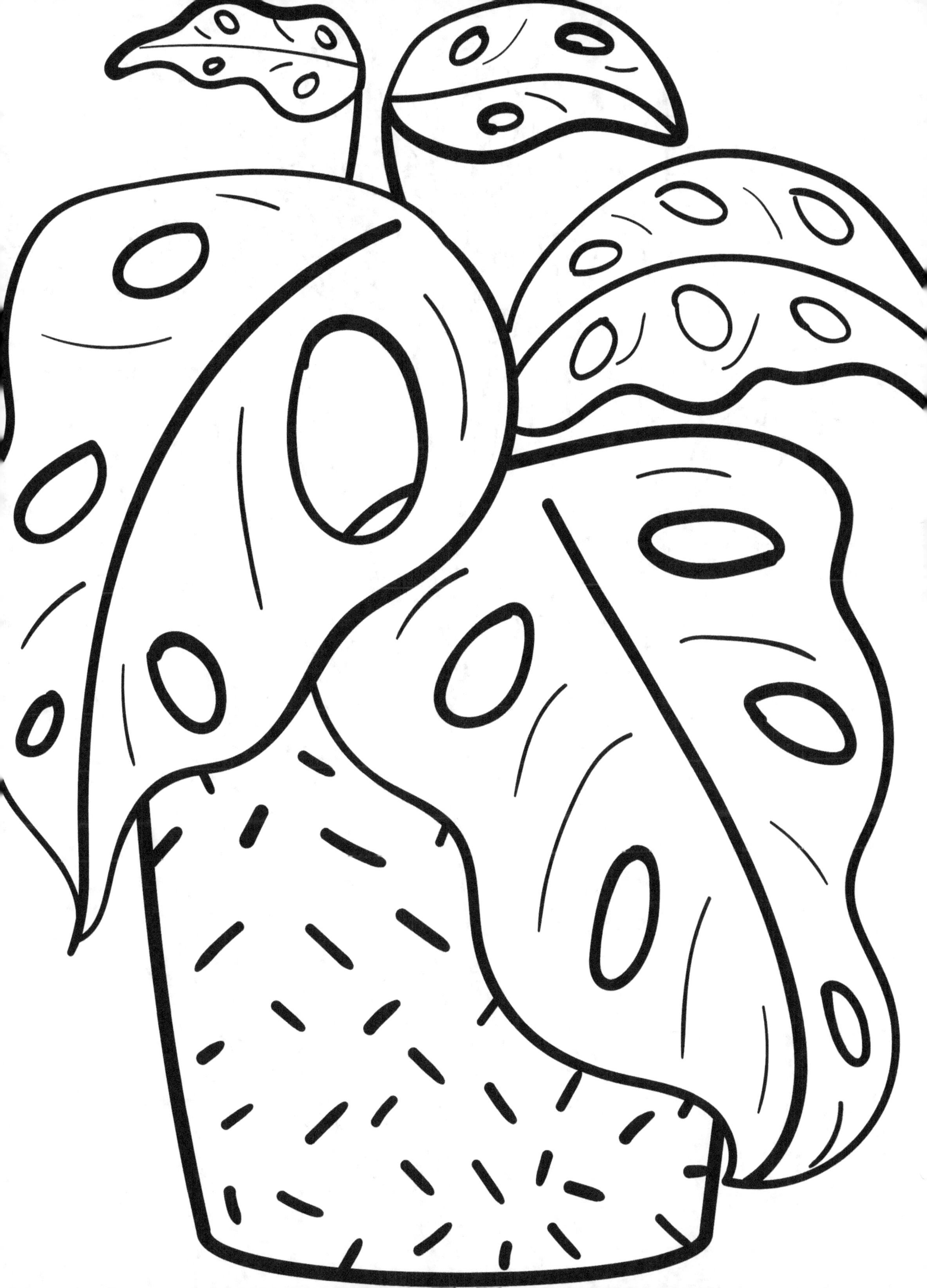

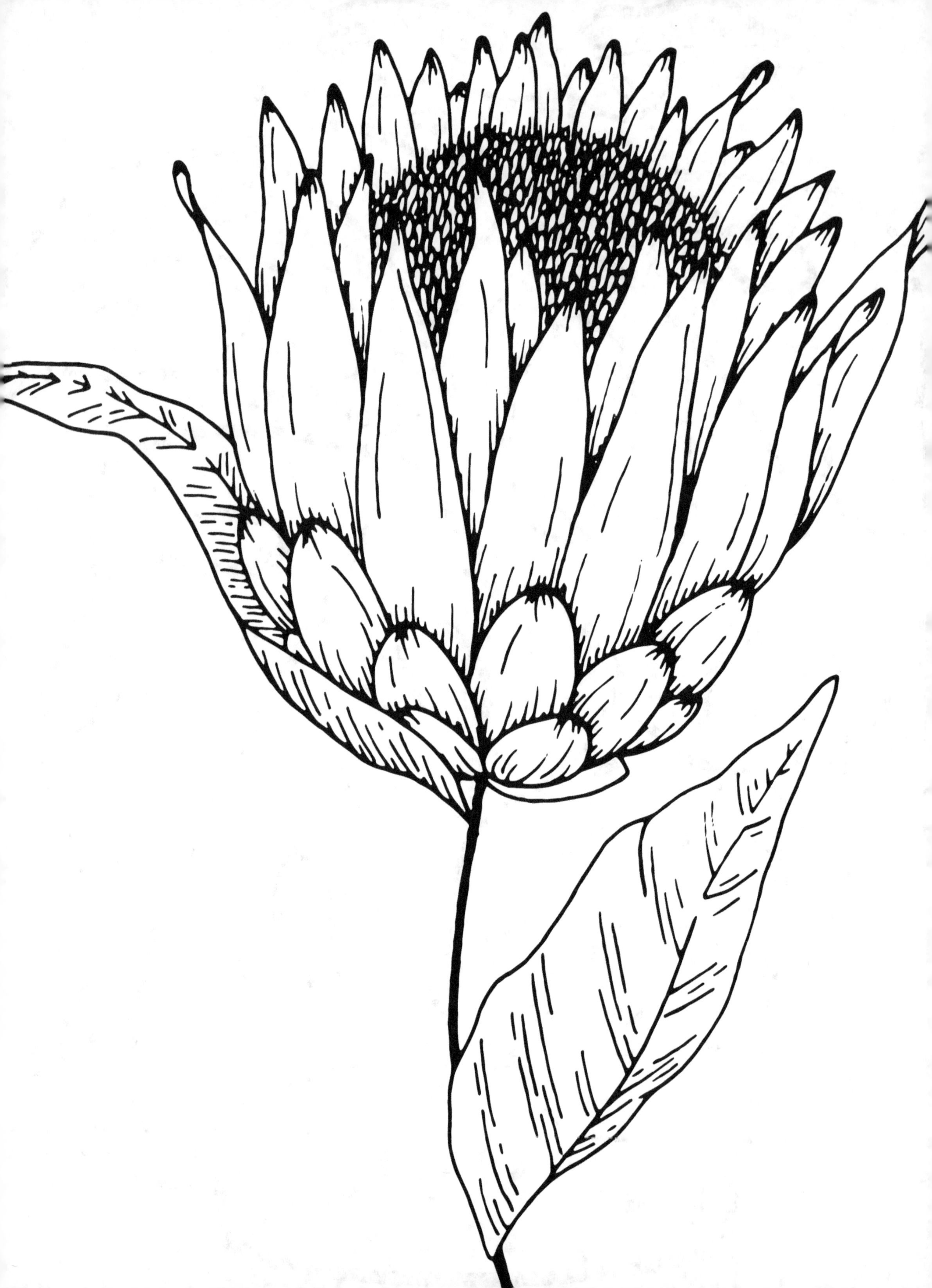

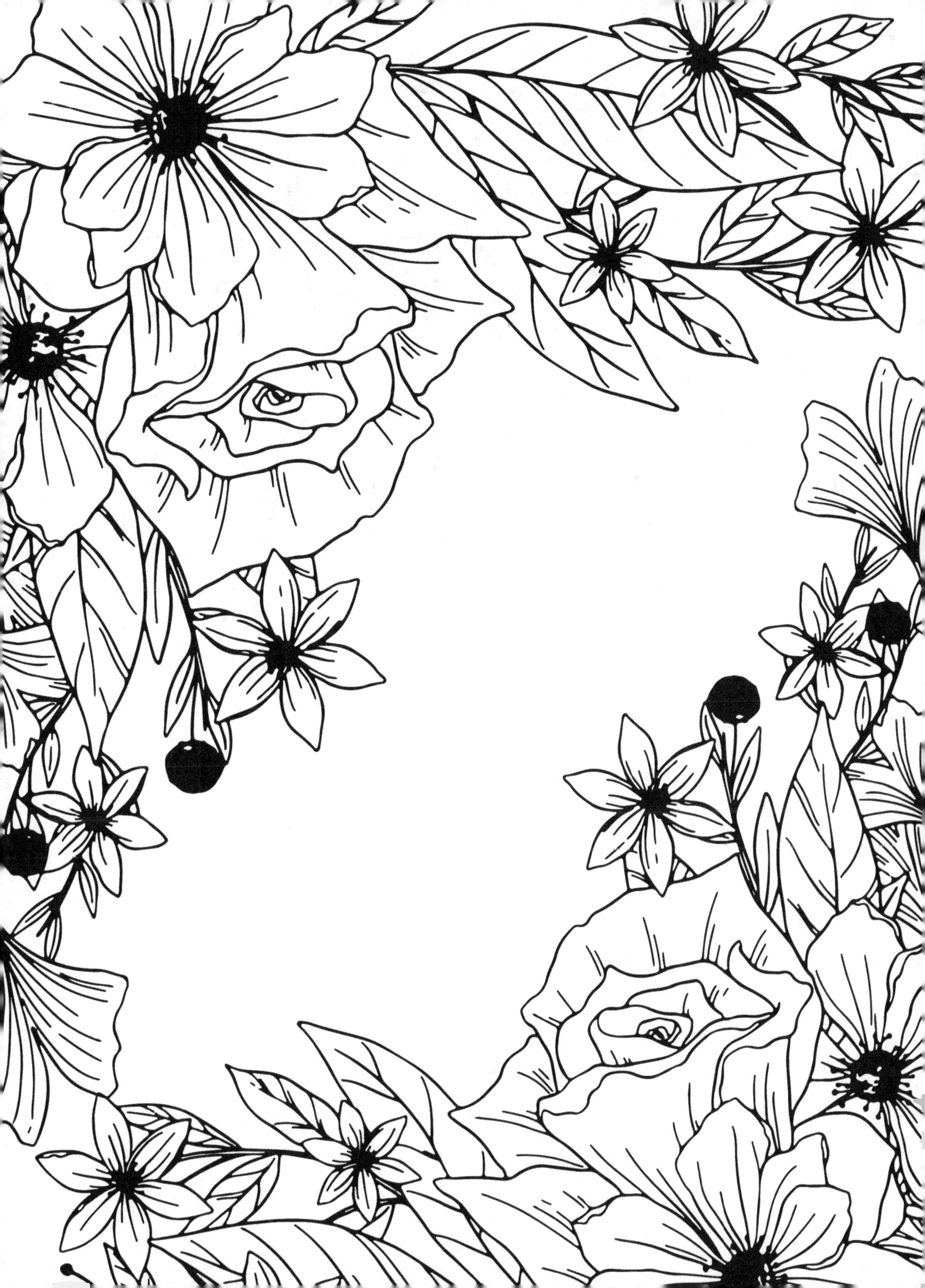

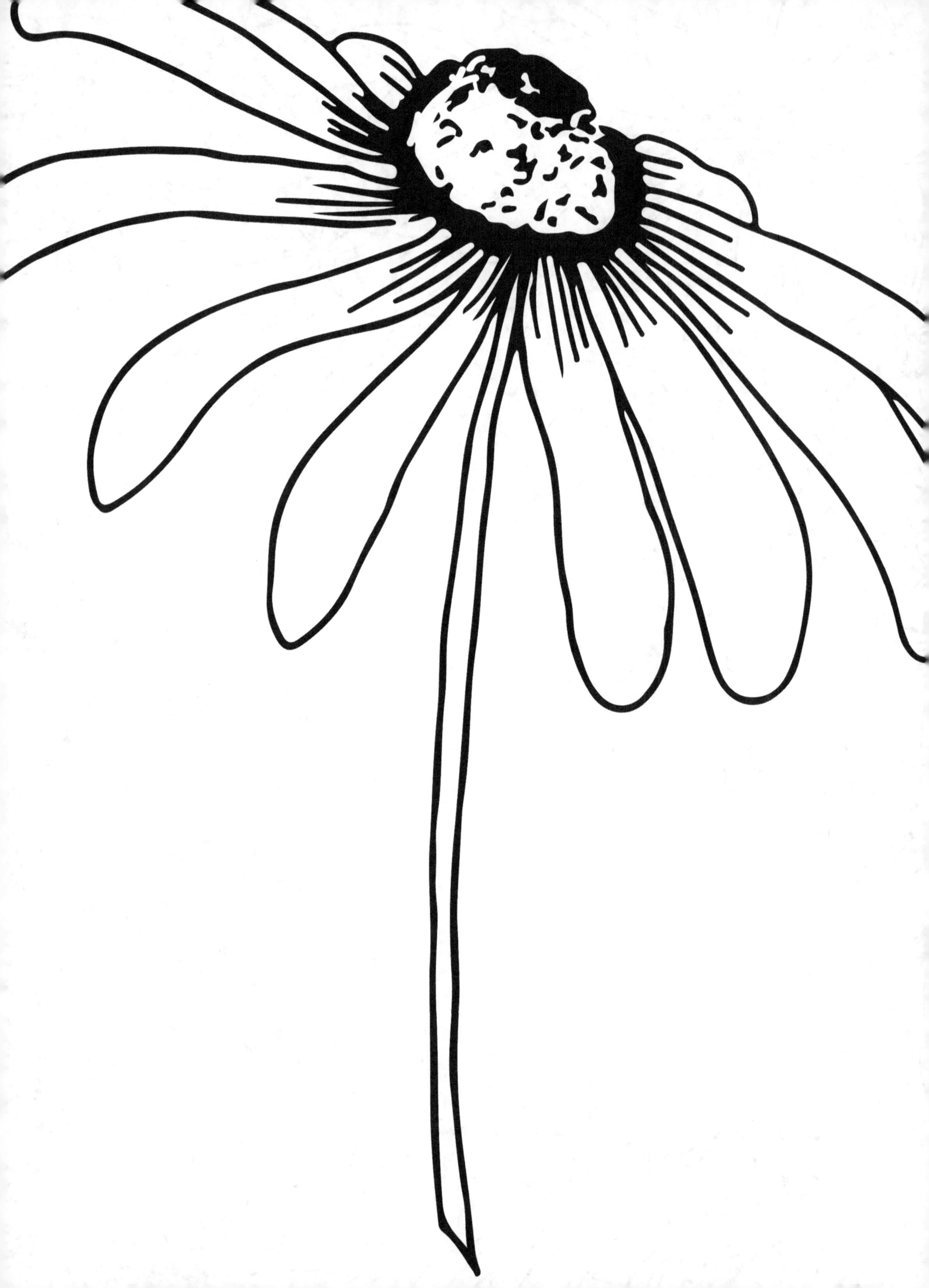

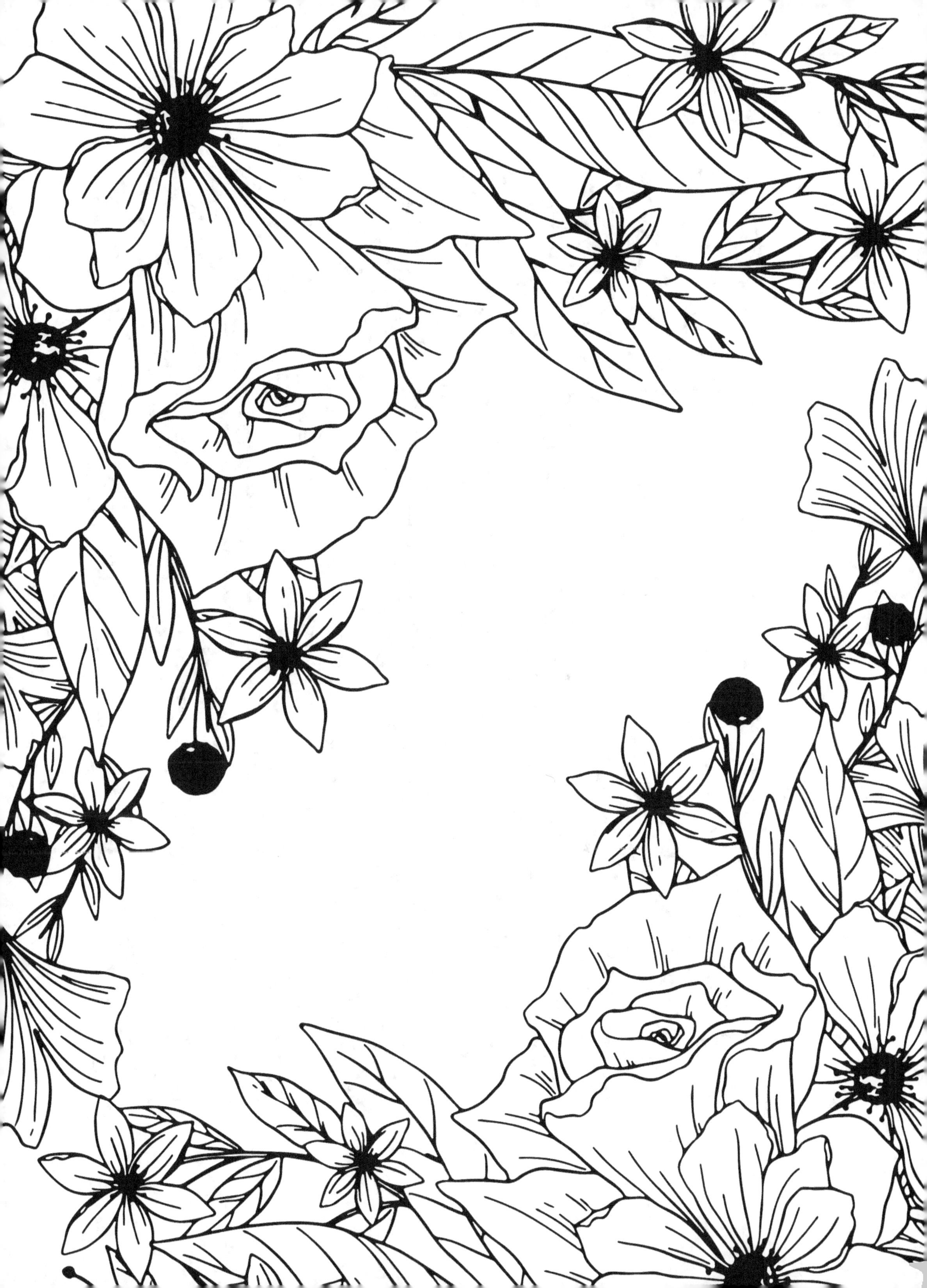

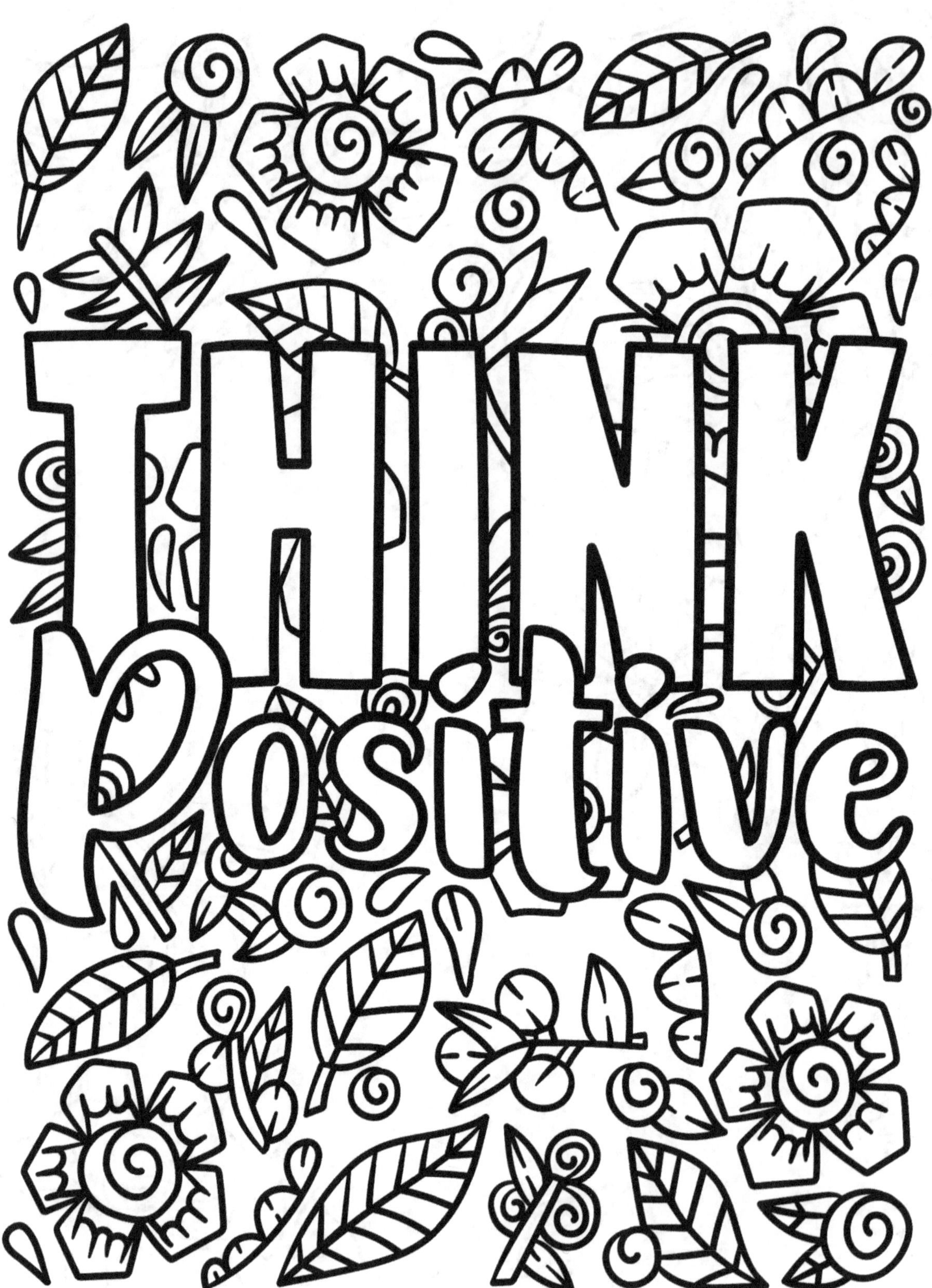
THINK
Positive

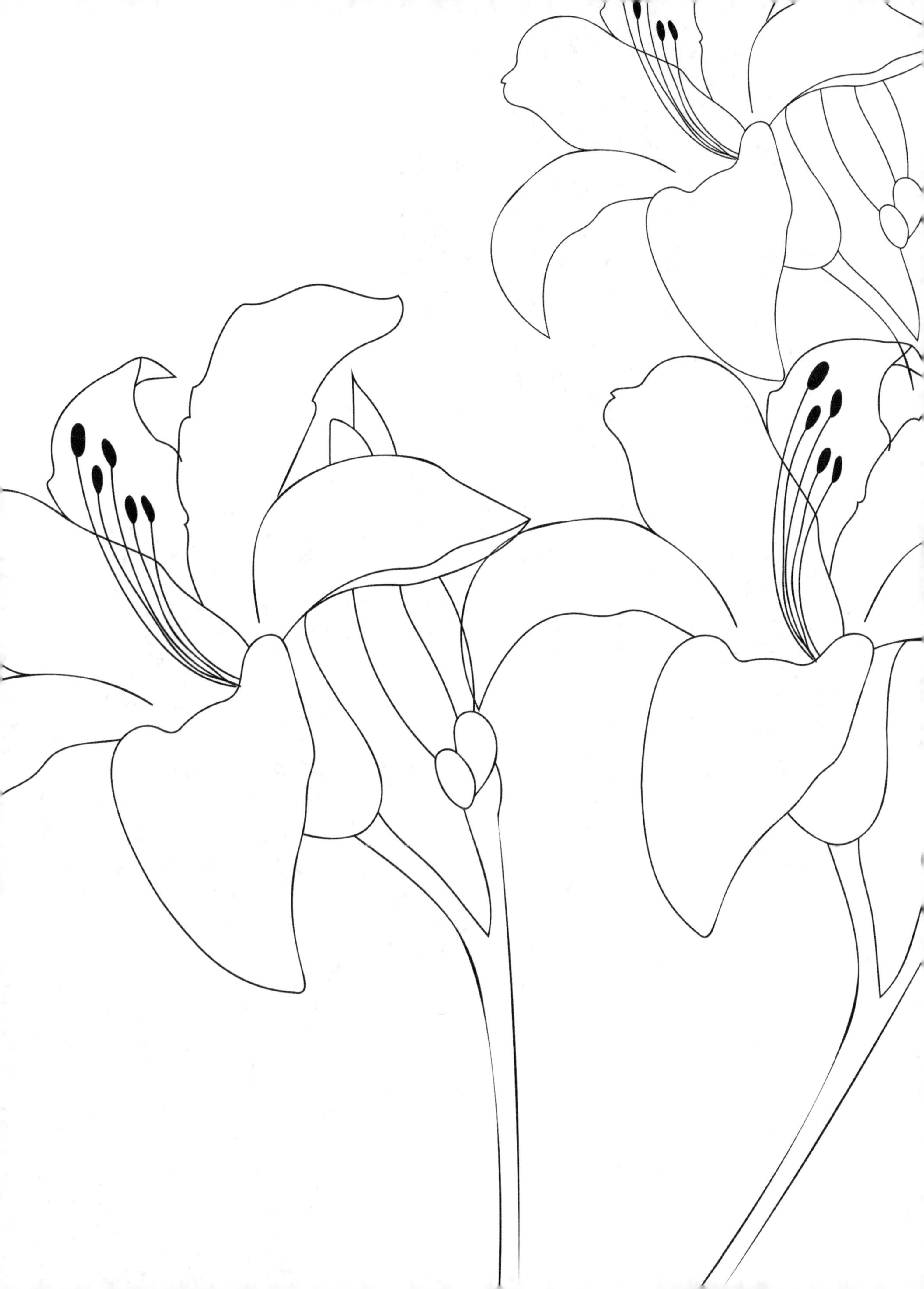

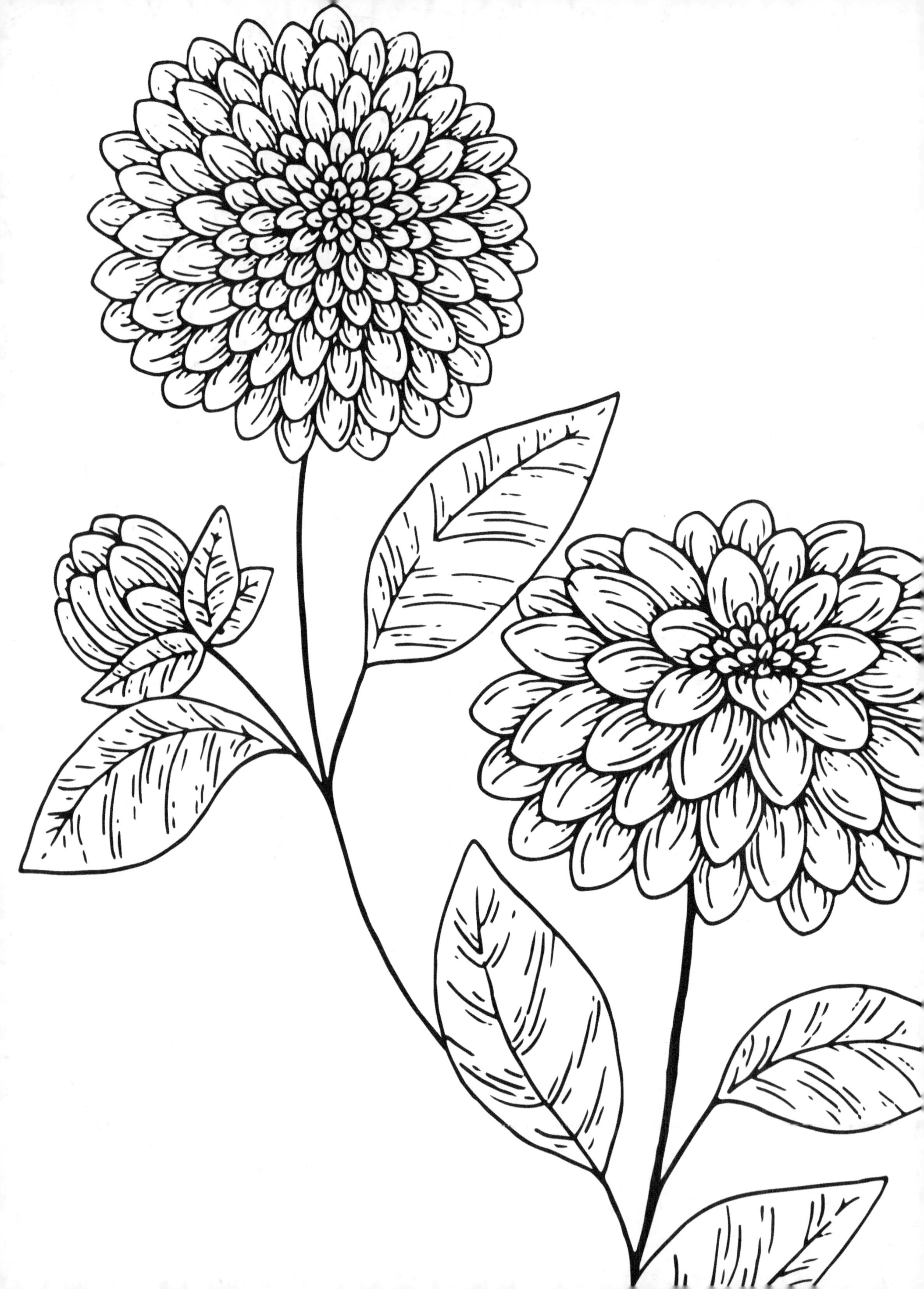

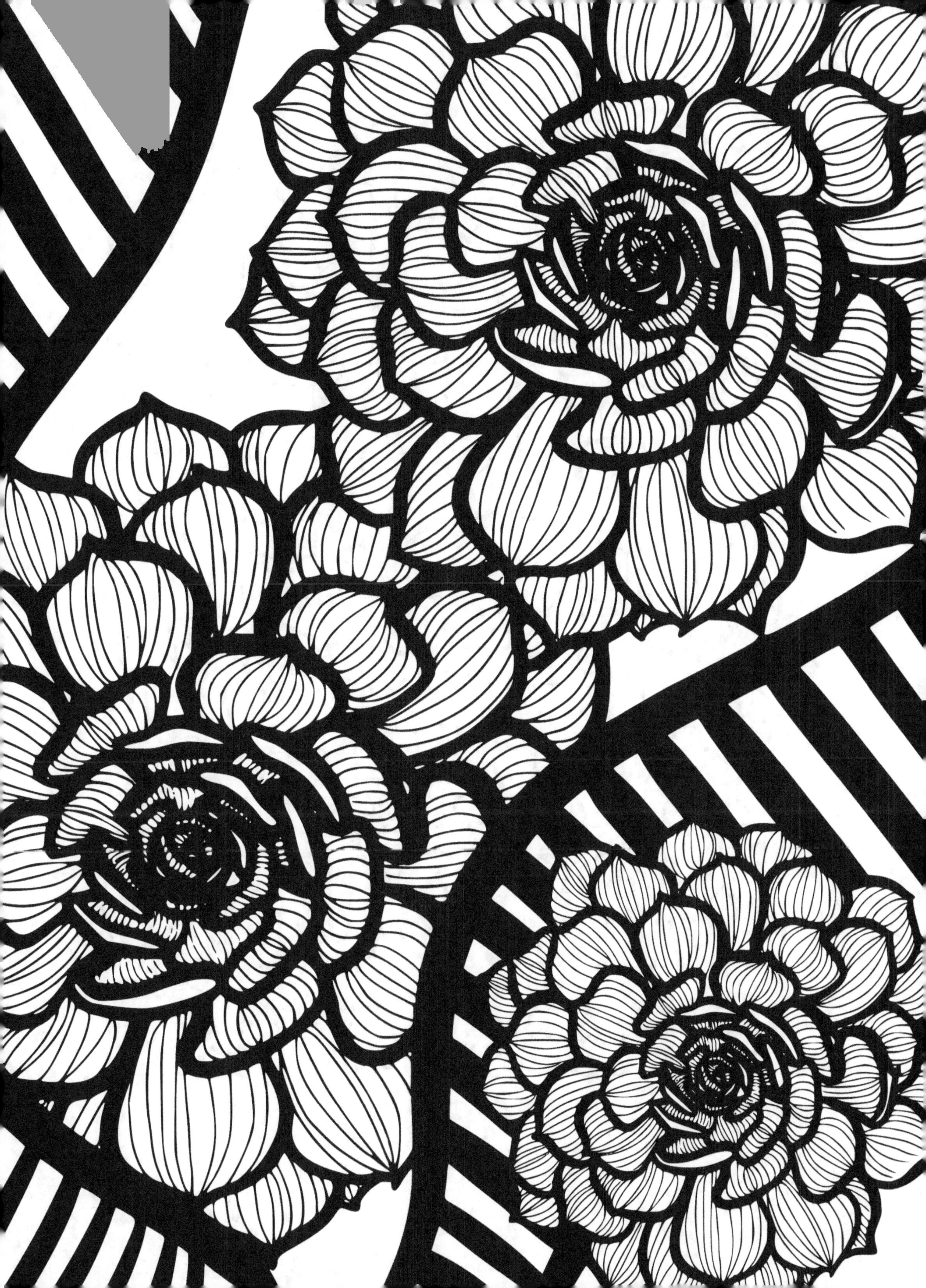

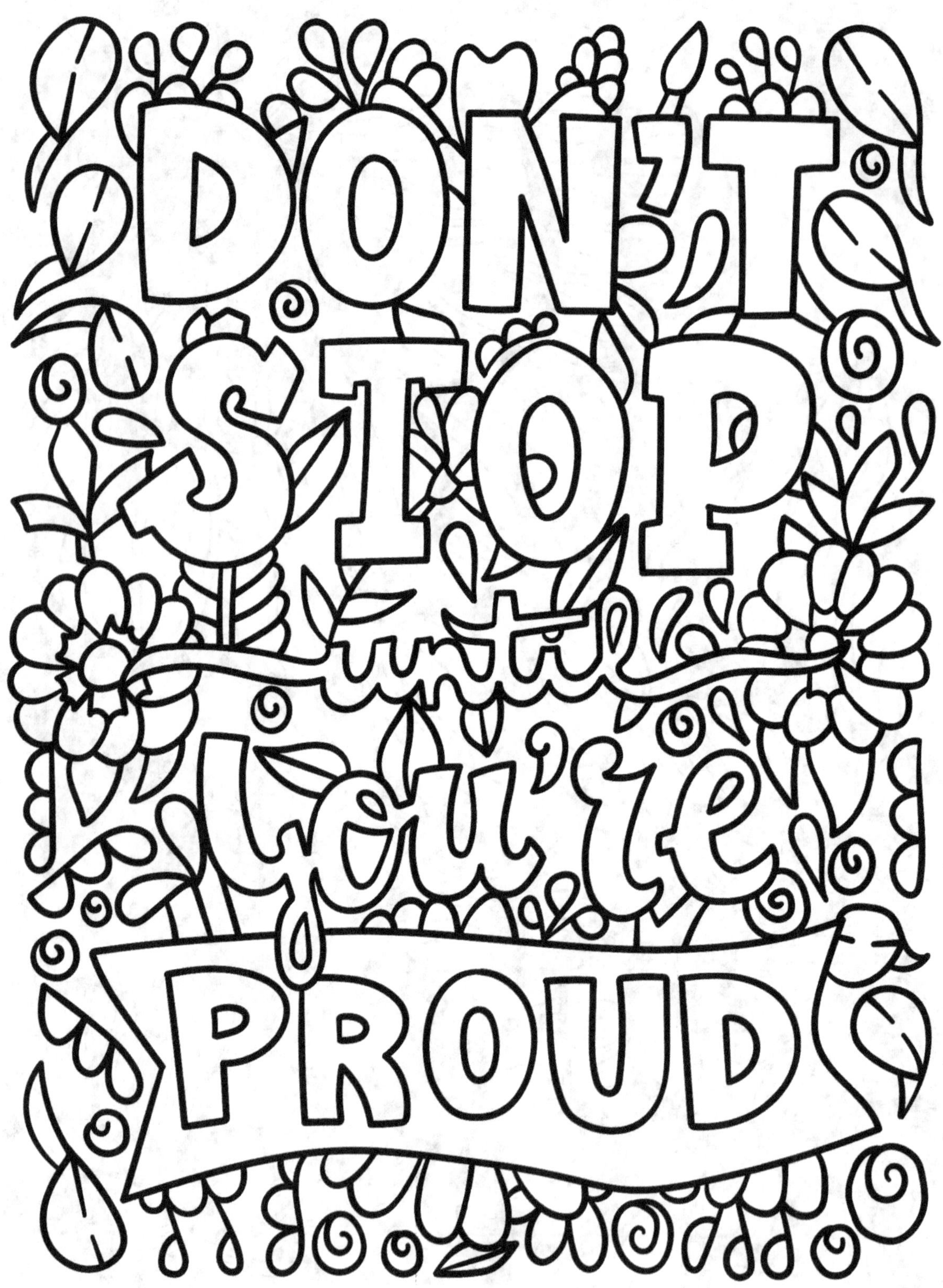

DON'T
STOP
until
you're
PROUD

www.ingramcontent.com/pod-product-compliance
Lightning Source LLC
Chambersburg PA
CBHW081743280726
48660CB00022B/3745